Lap-Band® Struggles

Revisit. Rethink. Revise.

Dr. Duc C. Vuong

This edition published by HappyStance Publishing

Print Edition ISBN-13: 978-0692650097

Print Edition ISBN-10: 0692650091

This book is intended for informational purposes only. This book does not offer medical advice, so nothing in it should be construed as medical advice. You should not act or rely on anything in this book or use it as a substitute for medical advice from a licensed professional. The content of this book may become outdated, especially due to the nature of the topics covered, which are constantly evolving. The information in this book is not guaranteed to be correct, complete, or timely. Certain sections of this book might have appeared in other written, audio, online, or video formats. Nothing in this book creates a doctor/patient relationship between the author and you, the reader. Although the author is a physician, he is most likely not your physician, unless he has seen you in his office as a patient. This book should not be used as a substitute to seeing your own physician.

Patient names and account details have been changed to protect patient identity. The scenarios are meant to be representative. Any similarities with your experience is only coincidental.

The original illustrations found in this book are only representative and not intended to be completely anatomically accurate. Variations in surgical technique exist among surgeons, so your surgeon might perform the surgery differently from what is depicted in the pictures. Please do not use the images as references. The opinions expressed in this book are derived through years of surgical experience, but may not represent the opinions of your surgeon. The statements made in this book do not indicate "rightness" or "wrongness" and because treatment modalities, medical literature, and technology constantly change they might become outdated. Please check with your surgeon or healthcare professional prior to making any medical decisions and do not depend solely on the contents of this book as your primary reference.

For my baby Chloe, whose beautiful spirit is so unbelievably close to its source.

Standardizations

Over the years, I've learned that for ease of reading, writing, and communicating, some standards should be set from the offset; therefore, I have decided on a few consistencies in this book. Approximately 75-80% of weight loss surgery patients are women, so when referring to patients, I will use the feminine form, such as "she" or "her." Likewise, since the vast majority of bariatric surgeons are men, I will use the masculine "he" or "his" when referring to surgeons. This is not meant in any way to exclude, judge, or offend anyone, but rather to reflect the current trends and provide consistency.

There are many different types of gastric bands worldwide, but since in the United States the Lap-Band, made by Allergan, now owned by Apollo, is the predominant market leader and therefore known to most patients, I will usually refer to it by name. What I write, however, applies to all brands of gastric bands.

The vertical sleeve gastrectomy will often be referred to as "the sleeve" or "gastric sleeve," and I will use "gastric bypass" the majority of the time when referring to Roux-en-Y gastric bypass. Sometimes duodenal switch will be shortened to "switch."

Contents

Introduction

"That men do not learn very much from the lessons of history is the most important of all the lessons of history." *– Aldous Huxley*

Because you are reading this book, you likely already know that much has changed in the past five years in bariatric surgery since the publication of my book, *Ultimate Lap-Band Success*. There has been a drastic decline in the percentage of gastric banding cases from about 50% of all bariatric surgeries in 2008 to about 10% in 2013. We've also seen the vertical sleeve gastrectomy ("sleeve" for short) rapidly rise to become the leading weight loss procedure in the U.S., and possibly worldwide. We have seen renewed interest in the duodenal switch and cautious optimism towards the mini-gastric bypass. New weight loss medicines have been approved for the first time in decades, and new technologies such as gastric balloons and endoscopic suturing exist, even if they are not (yet) readily available. Indeed, bariatric surgery is the most dynamic medical field of this decade.

Weight loss surgery has a long and sometimes checkered history. Surgery designed specifically for weight loss first emerged in the 1950's at the University of Minnesota. Through the years many procedures have come and gone, and a few have stood the test of time. The primary procedures now are gastric banding (Lap-Band), vertical sleeve gastrectomy (the sleeve), Roux-en-Y gastric bypass (RNYGB), and the biliopancreatic diversion with or without duodenal switch (BPD with or without DS). The last one is usually referred to as just duodenal switch or DS.

But many procedures had very short histories. A couple of these are the jejunoileal bypass (JIB) and the vertical banded gastroplasty. The jejunoileal bypass is highly malabsorptive because, while it keeps the stomach intact, it reroutes around much of the intestine, so nutrients are not taken up by the body in the normal amounts. Although weight loss with the JIB is good, many patients developed serious complications such as diarrhea, night blindness, osteoporosis, protein malnutrition, and liver failure. (Can you imagine being one of the patients who went blind? It certainly makes weight regain seem insignificant.) Consequently, the JIB is no longer recommended as a weight loss procedure. Often referred to as "stomach stapling," gastroplasty was designed in the early 1970s to be a safer alternative to the RYGBP and the JIB; it was the first purely restrictive operation performed for the treatment of obesity. The original gastroplasty involved stapling the stomach horizontally into a small partition, leaving only a small opening for food to pass from the smaller upper stomach pouch to the lower one. This form of gastroplasty resulted in very poor long-term weight loss and, after several attempted modifications, was eventually abandoned.

Why am I starting a book on gastric band revisions with a history lesson on bariatric surgery? The medical field has ample experience with forms of inadequate or "failed" weight loss surgeries besides gastric banding, *all* of which were much more radical and invasive than the band. You are not alone if you have had poor results with the Lap-Band, which are not necessarily due to a complication with the band itself, something you might or might not be doing, or a combination of both. By writing this book, my goal is to provide guidance on your current struggles with the Lap-Band—how to get back on track, what symptoms to watch for, and whether and how to decide to revise to another surgery. **This book is not intended to sway you, but rather to provide you with information.**

The 50-plus-year history with weight loss surgery has taught us that obesity is a complicated disease. Surgeons try to perform weight loss surgery uniformly, but we are becoming acutely aware that the procedures have varying effects on different people, and we are not sure why. We can perform exactly the same technical weight loss operation on two people, who by medical standards are similar, yet they can have very different results—one patient could do very well, but the other might not—and we are not sure why. Weight loss surgery is one of the very few medical fields in which surgical outcomes are highly dependent on postoperative patient behavior.

The American Medical Association (AMA) recognized obesity as a disease in 2013. Hence we are beginning to think of inadequate weight loss after surgery as an "incomplete treatment" rather than a "weight loss surgery failure."

"YOU ARE NOT A FAILURE, BUT RATHER HAVE INCOMPLETE TREATMENT OF YOUR DISEASE."

If your high blood pressure is not controlled with one medicine, your doctor adds a second antihypertensive, or even a third if needed. If your HA1c is not low enough, he gives you another diabetes medicine or adds insulin. He definitely does not call you a "failure." So why do we do this with obesity? Obesity is a complex condition, consisting of a multitude of factors, so to think that a one-time surgery could address all of the different aspects is a little like thinking that one type of insulin should work for all diabetics.

Once, after a Lap-Band to sleeve revision patient left my consultation, my clinic manager told me, "Mrs. Jones mentioned you said that the surgery won't work without fruits and vegetables. She got the impression that you don't believe in the surgery." Then my clinic manager asked, "You DO believe in weight loss surgery, don't you, Dr. V?!" I was taken aback by this question, since after all I *am* a bariatric surgeon who has written several books on the benefits of weight loss surgery.

After some contemplation, I answered my clinic manager's question:

"I BELIEVE IN OUR PROGRAM."

Weight loss surgery *alone* does not guarantee long term weight loss results, and we therefore have an intensive program in my practice. Like other devastating diseases, obesity has ramifications beyond physical health—it takes a toll on your emotions, relationships, and finances. Because my comprehensive bariatrics program focuses more on the psychological and emotional struggles of obesity than on the surgery itself, I have become known as the "Support Surgeon." After patients complete all of the insurance requirements (which include monthly dietary visits and mandatory pre-operative weight loss), they come on average 8-10 weeks in a row to educational groups that I lead. These are educational groups, not support groups, in which I teach them about the surgery, life with the surgery, and appropriate lifestyle changes. We also try to answer deeper questions like, *why do you make the choices you do? Why are you angry with your mother after all of these years? Who are you and what were you meant to do with your life?* It's through the insights gleaned in these groups that I've become intimate with the struggles of weight loss surgery patients. These regular educational group sessions supplement the normal follow-up visits that take place every three to six months. In my opinion, *optional* monthly support group meetings are not frequent enough, because if a patient misses one meeting, she will go two months without any support.

Because I interact so frequently with my patients, I am able to identify inadequate treatment early. Some may need more frequent follow-up care. Some may benefit from medically-supervised meal-replacements and diet pills. Why hang everything on the belief that a surgery alone should be sufficient, all while the number of revisions is steadily climbing? I also teach my patients to adopt a primarily pescatarian diet, which consists mostly of fresh fruits and vegetables, beans, whole grains, tofu, fish, and seafood. I am also readily accessible to my patients through email, Facebook, Periscope, and other social media. Without these non-surgical aspects, weight loss surgery has a high failure rate, possibly 30-50%, especially for those with a BMI (body mass index) above 50. So yes, I *do believe in the efficacy of weight loss surgery* to affect short-term change, but long-term happiness is dependent on much more.

"WEIGHT LOSS SURGERY IS AN OPPORTUNITY, NOT A GUARANTEE"

From my long experience in working with Lap-Band patients, I have learned that many patients do not receive the preoperative education or postoperative care needed to be successful with the band. (Whether it is available or not is a different matter.) Too many patients never return to their clinics for an adjustment (which makes the procedure about as effective as never having the surgery) or do not receive the proper number of adjustments to feel the promised sense of satiety. The reasons for this are many—convenience, cost, distance, loss of insurance, good intentions but lack of follow-through, and a host of others. More often, however, I have found that the opposite is true—band patients are often too tight for too long. Many chase the idea that they need to be tighter, without understanding that this causes many of the problems with the band. I think this is a consequence of the "my band is a tool" mentality. I talk about this in the next chapter, but briefly, it becomes too easy either 1) to ignore the tool and not use it correctly or 2) to depend too much on the tool.

I have a different concept. In my clinic, we refer to the weight loss surgery as a "new baby." It doesn't matter if it's a baby band, sleeve, bypass, duodenal switch, or whatever might come next. Think of a new mother who has just brought home her newborn baby for the first time. She loves it, caresses it, and holds it with such tenderness.

"YOU MUST TREAT YOUR BABY WITH LOVE AND TENDERNESS."

We do everything to make sure our babies have the best starts and opportunities available by giving them the very best. What types of teenagers our babies grow into—whether good or mischievous, kind or troubled, thankful or selfish—depend not on the number of years that have passed but rather on the seeds that were planted when they were young. This is also true of your weight loss surgery baby. How successful you are with your weight loss journey will be heavily dependent on how you treat your new baby after surgery. So you must give it the best. You must always be kind and treat it with loving tenderness.

Dr. George Fielding, a renowned weight loss surgeon from New York University, has been very successful keeping weight off with his Lap-Band. I asked him to give his input regarding the band, and here is what he had to say:

> "It'll be 16 years this December 2015 since I made the decision that changed my life forever. I was fat, sick, and sick of it. Actually, I was scared I was going to die. In one year, I'd ended up on 11 new medications. I was doing a lot of bariatric surgery in 1999, and realized that I was as fat and sick as most of my patients. I looked in the mirror and told myself it was time. I [decided to have] a Lap-Band. I had it on a Thursday, flew one thousand miles home on Friday, went back to work on Monday, and was never the same again. I had been ruled by hunger, and a restless, insatiable, constant urge to eat for my whole life. I'd lost a lot of weight, 60 to 80 pounds, numerous times, but always put it back on. Since that December day in 1999, I've lost about 120 pounds, and have kept it off. I love cooking. I love going to restaurants. I collect recipes. I cook with the herbs, vegetables and eggs my wife grows. I just don't eat a lot, and I'm not hungry. I'm still 210 pounds at 6 feet tall.
>
> I, more than most, know that having a band isn't easy. I've performed about 9000 Lap-Band surgeries. I've seen the struggles people have. It all boils down to eating slowly above all else. Yes, it's tight in the morning. Yes, some days food I ate yesterday can be difficult today, especially if I'm tired or cranky. I've learned that you can't live your life as if you don't have a band. It will win every time if you eat fast. I've learned that you can't have it both ways. For the band to work, you have to eat slowly. Very slowly. I would rather eat slowly and stay the way I am, than be able to eat fast and be fat."

Keeping off 120 pounds for 16 years is quite an achievement with any surgery! Dr. Fielding's story should serve as a reminder of what is possible with the band if it is used correctly.

I hope that as you read this book, you will learn the anatomy and physiology required to make the gastric band work successfully and some of the things that could derail your weight loss success with the band. More importantly, I hope you will learn the mindset necessary to make *any* weight loss surgery successful. Armed with this new knowledge, you can make an informed decision either to revise your band or to make the band work for you **so that you can live the life you want to live and become the person you want to be.**

For the latest in free health tips and videos, please visit Dr. Duc Vuong (The Support Surgeon) at www.UltimateGastricSleeve.com or follow him on Facebook.

1

"The Lap-Band Is Just a Tool"

"Surgery is only 1 point in a continuum. Today is the day you need to start, not wait for the surgery to change your lifestyle.

– Dr. Eric DeMaria, Bariatric Surgery Pioneer

"The Lap-Band is just a tool." Right after you had your surgery, you were likely highly motivated to be a healthier eater and more active person. The pounds probably dropped off quickly in those first weeks, and you were excited to be able to fit into smaller sizes. Coworkers, friends, and family were all impressed with the changes they saw and regularly complimented your new lifestyle. All of this positive attention gave you not only a morale boost, but also constant reinforcement. Sometimes, it may have been hard learning how to eat, what to eat, and when to eat, but overall, it was pretty easy to lose weight. You ate a small amount of food and felt pressure, (which you thought was the same as fullness.)

Now the surgery and that initial excitement are in the distant past. The same small amount of food is not as satisfying. Hunger returns more frequently and hangs around longer. Everyone has gotten used to the New You and nobody comments on how great you look, except occasionally when you bump into an old acquaintance. Walking way across the parking lot to your car and taking the stairs do not make you sweat like they used to, and remembering what your surgeon said, you now feel even more pressure to include more exercise into your day. But you have deadlines at work, increasing family obligations, fun social activities planned, and a lot else going on. You need to focus on so many aspects of your life right now that cooking a fresh meal takes a backseat to other items on your long list of things to do. And did I mention how hungry you are? Since you've shifted away from making your "new" lifestyle your number one priority, your weight loss probably has slowed or stopped. Perhaps you even regained a few pounds. One day you look in the mirror and think, "Oh no. The Old Me is returning. What's happening here? Is my tool broken?"

All tools need maintenance—so too does the Lap-Band. Even with proper maintenance, all tools will eventually break down—so too will the Lap-Band. If you are not happy with your band, then you might fit into one or more of the categories below:

- Lost weight and had a complication with the Band, such as band slip or erosion.
- Lost weight but at the cost of vomiting, mucus production, and a poor social life.
- Lost some weight with the band but not as much as you had hoped.
- Never lost weight with the band.

John's Story

John had had his band for over two years, and his life had changed. He dropped from 450 to 275 pounds. Though technically still overweight at 6 feet tall, he was much happier—he had found a new job working in construction, made more money, had a new girlfriend, and took road trips he hadn't previously been able to manage. He was jovial and often the "class clown" during education group, as well as kind and well-liked.

One night, I got a call from John, who was struggling with his band. He hadn't been able to keep anything down for a couple of days, and even worse, he was starting to have abdominal pain. I instructed him to go to our local hospital, where I performed an x-ray called a barium swallow that showed that his band had slipped. Due to his abdominal pain, I decided it was best to act quickly; I took him to the operating room that night.

It was the first time I had to remove a Lap-Band, and it was nothing like what had been described in all the courses I took. While it is easy for me now, at that time in the middle of the night, the surgery was intense. The stomach tissues were very inflamed—nothing like anything I had ever seen before—and I had trouble even finding the band. After a couple of hours, I was able to take out the band safely and make sure that John's stomach tissues would survive.

When I talked to John's parents in recovery and showed them the pictures of what I had found—a slipped band with compromised stomach tissues—I was overcome by a sense that I had let him down. I knew that statistically he was most likely going to regain all of his weight, but I held on to the hope that maybe his hard work, knowledge, and dedication to the new lifestyle would be enough to stop the weight regain.

I have lost touch with John. Maybe he thought he had let me or his friends in support group down. Maybe he had regained some weight and was embarrassed. Maybe he was upset with the band or with me. I wish I could tell him that I miss him, that it was not his fault, that his weight-loss journey was not over. I wish I could tell him that his weight loss success was due to his persistence and determination, not solely to his band.

Patricia's Story

Patricia was a young single mom. She worked hard and was disciplined with her time management. She had the Lap-Band placed when she reached her heaviest weight of about 250 pounds. Through dedication, planning, and regular exercise, she dropped to 125 pounds and a normal BMI of 22. She was very happy with this result and content with her life. In order to complete her transformation, she decided to get an abdominoplasty, also known as a "tummy tuck." She recovered well from the surgery without any complications.

About six months after her plastic surgery, Patricia called my office to say that she was having trouble keeping any food down. A barium swallow x-ray showed that she had a small slip. I removed her band's fluid and placed her on liquids for two weeks. After a repeat barium swallow indicated that the band remained slipped, I added another two weeks of the liquid diet.

I wasn't too concerned, because on all accounts, Patricia was very successful with her band. At her one-month follow-up appointment, I was surprised to find her distraught, convinced that she would regain the weight. "I've worked too hard for this body, Dr. V," she said. I explained to her that her slip was very small and not symptomatic, so we could leave it deflated for a while. I explained that the band had done its job and that she was now a healthy weight, but she remained upset because she "could not use her tool." I explained that her "tool" was still in her and could possibly be reinflated later. I tried my best to convince her that it was her hard work and dedication that made her such a success, but she was overcome with the fear that she *could* regain weight and *could* lose control around food without her band being tight. At the end of our office visit, she agreed to see a psychologist familiar with obesity-related issues.

Amanda's Story

Amanda and her husband were newlyweds looking forward to starting a family. After years of not being able to conceive, Amanda became pregnant when she lost 100 pounds within a year after having the Lap-Band placed. I completely deflated her band, because she was suffering from terrible morning sickness. She delivered a healthy baby boy.

Amanda came back to my clinic when her son was one-year-old because she felt it was time to "get back on track," even though she weighed the same as when her band was deflated and was only 20 pounds from her goal weight. I performed the barium swallow in my office and everything looked fine at first. I had her swallow a little bit more, and in the next series of x-rays, a small bit of barium flowed over instead of through the band, suggesting a band erosion. I confirmed this with an endoscopy, a quick examination under sedation where a small camera passes down the throat into the stomach. Her Lap-Band needed to be removed and the hole in her stomach repaired.

When I told Amanda about her situation, she took it very well. Instead of taking her immediately to surgery (she was doing well clinically), I talked with her about attending my preoperative program to get the education my usual patients do. I felt that because she was so close to her goal weight, my preoperative and postoperative diet plan would probably get her to her goal. She agreed, stating that she felt the education and support was what she had been lacking the whole time.

****

What's the difference among these three stories? Why did John's band slip after tremendous weight loss? Despite having a healthy BMI, why did Patricia not believe that she was now "normal"? Why did Amanda accept the removal of her band while Patricia could not accept the temporary deflation of hers?

These stories and others resonate in my mind when I hear people call their weight loss surgery a "tool."

"WEIGHT LOSS SURGERY IS NOT JUST A TOOL."

Everyone seems to hammer (pun intended) the description of the surgery as a tool into patients' minds. "My Lap-Band (sleeve, bypass, etc…) is just a tool." **While the comparison has some merit, it is inadequate.** Many people have tool sheds full of very expensive equipment. They may have a riding lawnmower, a power blower, a lawn edger, a weed-eater, etc…but yet they may still hire a professional landscaping company. Or they pay the teenage boy from across the street $25 to mow the lawn using an old broken down push mower. It's not enough to know that you have a "tool" at your disposal—you have to be willing to pick it up and use it, and not just once in awhile, but all of the time! You should also be taught the proper use of the tool. You have to maintain a tool, but many owners do not, instead letting their tools rust away or gather cobwebs. And if your tool needs professional fixes, not all repairmen are the same. A mechanic might not make the best repairs or even know what to do. Worse, he might not even admit that he doesn't know exactly what to do. All of this is a set up for failure.

Instead, think

"MY WEIGHT LOSS SURGERY IS NOT A TOOL, BUT RATHER AN OPPORTUNITY."

Tools will eventually break down, but it's up to us to make the most of our opportunities.

Here is the analogy I prefer to describe the role of weight loss surgery: Remember the old-fashioned Big-Top Circuses? Remember the giant cannon and the man who climbs into it? Imagine the daredevil being shot out of the cannon, flying across the Big-Top, and landing safely on a large net on the other side.

Many patients think that the weight loss surgery is the cannon—the my-surgery-is-a-tool mentality. They think that as long as they get into the cannon, it will shoot them far into the air, and they will go soaring easily to their destination. But the surgery is NOT the cannon. The surgery is instead the NET on the other side that catches them. It keeps them from falling too far and getting hurt. So what then is the cannon?

"YOU ARE THE CANNON!"

You will determine how far you will go. Your attitude, determination, and persistence—not the weight loss surgery—will get you to your goals. As the net, the surgery will catch you if you fall, but how high you fly and how far you go are completely dependent on YOU. You have ALWAYS been the cannon. Your gains, and also your losses, have always been the result of your actions and decisions, not the band's. If you are struggling with weight loss, then most likely, it is not the band that that needs fixing or fine-tuning, but rather you.

You might be thinking, "No way Dr. V! I've done everything right!" Are you sure? Maybe in the beginning you did, but how about lately? Weight regain has to do with something you are eating but shouldn't be, or something you should be eating but aren't. It is about running when you are still walking. It is about salads not protein shakes. It is about laughing and loving and not worrying about your sick mother or your possible separation from your spouse. There is ALWAYS something that can get you off track, and it is easy to look to the Band as the problem. In the first story, John did not come to see me when he had obstructive symptoms and was vomiting on an almost daily basis. A partial deflation could have possibly prevented his slip. In Patricia's story, she could not see that even though her band was temporarily out of service, it was her mindset that needed fixing. There are definitely times when the band is broken—it is too tight, has slipped, or has eroded and causes the patient to vomit daily or have pain when eating. Then there are times when the patient is broken. Perhaps she demands a fill because she doesn't feel any restriction, but a barium swallow shows that the barium is obstructed in her esophagus because the band is too tight. There are times when the patient complains of obstruction and "only ice cream" will go down, but the barium passes easily through the band. Obesity is physically complex, but the workings of the mind are even more complex.

So step back and reassess the problem. Try to answer,

"Is my Band failing me, or am I failing my Band?"

Then take action.

Summary and Tips: "My Lap-Band is MORE than just a TOOL."

1) A Tool needs regular maintenance.

a. The last time I saw my surgeon was ______________________________.

b. The last time I had a barium swallow was ______________________________.

c. The last time I had an EGD was ______________________________.

2) My Lap-Band is a safety net.

a. My dream weight loss goal is to weigh ______________________pounds.

b. If I could not get down to my dream weight loss goal, I'd be happy if I weighed ____ pounds. This is my happy weight.

c. If I could not get down to my happy weight, I'd think the surgery was a success if I weighed ____ pounds or if I ______________________________.

3) I am the CANNON!

a. To get down to my goal weight, I will ______________________________.
(example keep a food journal, go see my surgeon, start daily exercises, read more about nutrition, learn to meditate.)
b. I currently weigh ______________pounds.
c. I will weigh ________________pounds by ____________________ (date.)
d. I've called my surgeon and my next appointment is ________________.

2

The Truth About Hunger

"Your IDEA of happiness might be the biggest barrier to your true happiness." *– Thich Nhat Hanh, Buddhist monk*

Patients have many reasons to explain the return of their lost pounds, but the one I hear and read about the most is Hunger. "I'm getting hungry again! What do I do?!" Many patients think they would be happy if they never felt hungry again. Americans tend to think that they should never be hungry and always be full. Have you ever asked where this notion came from? Continual fullness is the promise of every diet and every weight loss surgery, isn't it? "Sprinkle this powder on your food, and you will get full on less." "Eat this bar, and you won't be hungry between meals." "Place this band around your stomach, and you will be full after eating a small meal." "Have this surgery and you won't get hungry between meals."

Many preoperative patients say, "Dr. Vuong, I don't want to be hungry anymore," or "I can't wait until I'm no longer hungry!" They are surprised when I tell them what I'm about to tell you:

"IT IS NATURAL TO BE HUNGRY. IT IS UNNATURAL TO BE FULL."

I have a lot of experience with hunger. I spent six months in a refugee camp in Thailand as a young child. Most people who meet me don't realize this because even though I am Asian, I don't speak English with an accent. They assume I was born in America, but I was not. My father and I were some of the "boat people" you might have heard about after the Vietnam War ended. My father made a daring escape with me in his arms one dark night in a little boat full of people. We ended up coming ashore at a refugee camp in Thailand, where there were lots of skinny, dark-haired refugees and very little food. So I am no stranger to hunger. I could have easily allowed myself to be controlled or defined by my hunger. But I didn't. Instead I chose to embrace my hunger as an experience that I had to go though (and continually go through) in order to be the person I am today (and will be tomorrow.)

Whenever I get hungry, I eat. Hunger pangs are my body's way of telling me that it needs nourishment. I appreciate that simple luxury now—the gift of knowing that if I am hungry, I can easily find nourishing food. But there is a reason why Thanksgiving only comes around once a year. It is unnatural to feel "stuffed." The problem is that many Americans want it to be Thanksgiving at every meal. They want to feel full every time they eat and never to be hungry between meals. This is just not realistic. It is not how our bodies have evolved.

Unfortunately, the field of bariatrics has convinced many Americans that weight loss surgery will miraculously eliminate one's sensation of hunger. In my experience, this is not true long term. I am very happy if my patients eat until they are satisfied at mealtimes and are able to resist snacking between meals. Most snacks in America are not good for you because they are "quick and easy." Snacks are conveniently located down the hallway at the nearest vending machine. Sometimes, they are not even that far away, right in our own desk drawers or on the countertop. We have to learn to resist this snacking temptation. Snacking, for the most part, is an American invention. The rest of the world typically does not snack, and the countries that do often have obesity rates similar to those of the United States. Even if you are a diabetic, I strongly recommend that you minimize your snacking. Except for the occasional post-workout refueling, snacking does very little for you except to increase your daily caloric intake. The truth about hunger and weight loss is:

"IN ORDER TO LOSE WEIGHT, YOU MUST REDUCE YOUR CALORIC INTAKE; IN ORDER TO REDUCE YOUR CALORIC INTAKE, YOU MUST ALLOW YOURSELF TO BECOME HUNGRY."

To reduce your food consumption, you must eat more nutritious foods and understand their calorie density. **I don't like to focus on calories, so I tell my patients to pack in the most nutrition per bite most of the time!** If you eat French fries every day, it is no wonder that you are tired all of the time. As you lose weight and become more active, your body will need more energy to keep going. It will need better fuel than what it has gotten in the past. The body's fuel gauge for energy relies on REAL HUNGER (not pseudo-hunger borne of boredom, stress, or proximity to snacks), and the body's fuel is REAL FOOD, which is fresh fruits and vegetables and Mother Earth's other provisions.

I teach my patients to figure out whether they are really hungry or whether they are feeling psychological hunger. Real hunger manifests itself with measurable physical changes—decreased blood sugar, weakness, sweating, jitteriness, dizziness, etc. Psychological hunger does not come with these physical changes (even though your stomach may still rumble), but rather is triggered by the thought, sight, or smell of food. This is often situational. For example, you might develop cravings when a food commercial comes on during your favorite TV show, your husband reheats last night's pizza, or you walk by a cookie stand that triggers a childhood memory of a time you spent with your grandmother.

If you feel hungry, make sure it is really hunger that you are feeling. **Drinking a big glass of water may drive away psychological hunger.** I drink water all day long, especially around lunch time and at work. Assess whether it is an appropriate time to be hungry and whether you might be in a situation that could trigger psychological hunger. **Brush your teeth.** The strong flavor of toothpaste will often distract you from food thoughts. If you put yourself in a different situation—you **turn off the TV** and go outside or you move away from the smells of baking, for example—you might find that you're not "hungry" a few minutes later.

A "meal" is something very different for a weight loss surgery patient. Sometimes, this is hard for patients to recognize or understand. A lot of my patients think they are eating too much (maybe this is because I have them practice eating from a little saucer of food). After reviewing their meals, I am happy to point out to most of my patients that they are actually eating the right amount of food! It is just more than what they THOUGHT they should eat. Sometimes, I point out that they should increase the texture of what they eat so the food will stay longer in the gastric pouch. Maybe they are scared to move away from mushy tuna fish salad and have been avoiding chicken or meat for fear that it would get stuck. The Texture Scale is useful in these situations. I have included a summary of the Texture Scale in Appendix A.

Here is a not-too-uncommon scenario from a gastric band patient:

Mary's Story

Mary was about 2 months postop and was doing very well, losing weight at a steady pace. A week after her first adjustment, she complained that she was hungry all the time and thought the adjustment "didn't work." (Our clinic does explain that the average number of adjustments the first year is four or five but can vary from two to ten or more.) During our conversation, it became apparent that she was stressed because it was the one-year anniversary of her father's passing. Eventually, she said, "I don't even know why I am eating—I'm not even hungry when I do it…" We hugged, and I encouraged her to come to support group.

****

These highly emotional occasions will affect your weight loss journey, whether or not you want them to. No weight loss surgery will address such situations or will determine how you respond to them.

I tell my patients that whenever they get hungry, the first thing they should do is drink a big glass of water and wait 10 minutes. After 10 minutes, if they are still hungry, then they need to do a physical activity, like take a walk around the block. After that if they are still hungry and it is an appropriate meal time, they can eat. More often than not, they find that their "hunger" is not true hunger at all and is instead closely related to some emotion or condition, such as boredom, sadness, or loneliness. If you want to be successful in your weight loss journey, you must reevaluate your perception of hunger. **You must realize that hunger is not the enemy but a natural part of being you**. And in order to be successful, you must embrace all aspects of you.

Buddhist teaching tells us that whenever we feel hungry, we should be happy. This is because the only people who do not feel hungry are DEAD people. So whenever we feel hungry, we should be happy, because it means we are alive. Think to yourself,

"I'm hungry. This makes me happy. Hunger means I am alive. Without this hunger, I would not be."

My background as a hungry but happy child in a refugee camp gives me insights into food, health, and hunger that are not taught in medical school. My Asian heritage allows me to be more open to and confident in the ancient Eastern teachings that Western medicine often dismisses as fringe science at best and hocus-pocus at worst.

You need motivation to stick to your healthy choices and overcome your weight-loss "plateau." You can reach your happy weight, run a marathon, go back to school, get through the holidays without putting on pounds, or reach any of your other goals. You have the answers to your struggles. The trick is unlocking them, and introspection is the key that will open up this treasure chest. Start by thinking about all you have accomplished since your Lap-Band surgery, in terms of both your health and the rest of your life. **Give yourself proper credit for these accomplishments and then resolve to accomplish even more.** Start by setting a new goal. Make it a small, achievable goal, like increasing your daily water intake to 10 bottles. Then set another goal. And another goal, and so on, and so on. This will set the ball in motion.

If you perpetually believe that controlling your hunger is your "biggest hurdle" or "most difficult challenge," then what are you going to do when life really takes a whack at you? When you are laid off from your job, when a hurricane destroys your house, when your spouse leaves you for another? You and only you control your body, because you and only you can control your mind. And your mind controls everything. So don't fill your mind with small, trifling thoughts that don't accomplish much.

Remember, you are the cannon. How far you go, how high you fly, and how much you achieve are not determined by how many grams of protein you consume every day, but rather by your emotional and mental fortitude. The American Medical Association in 2013 recognized that obesity is a disease. I agree with this, except I would add that

"Obesity is primarily a mental illness. The war against obesity will be won or lost in the fields of your mind, not on your dinner plate."

What shows up on your dinner plate is ultimately nothing more than a reflection of what is happening in your mind.

Summary and Tips: "I'm hungry and this makes me happy because it means I AM ALIVE."

1) It's natural to be hungry. It's unnatural to be full. Write down how you feel after you've eaten too much. I feel:

____

____

____

2) To lose weight, you must decrease your caloric intake. To decrease your caloric intake, you must eat less. To eat less, you must allow yourself to get hungry. Write down why you are afraid of hunger.

____

____

____

3) When you feel hungry, first drink water. Then do an activity, such as go for a walk, garden, brush your teeth, use mouthwash. Write down what you will do next time you feel hungry.

____

____

____

4) When you feel hunger, think, "I'm hungry. This makes me happy because it means I'm alive." Write this phrase again.

____

____

____

5) Focus on all of the gains you've made instead of the fear that you might regain weight. Write down any health benefits you've had so far.

____

____

____

3

Weight Loss Plateau

"When we are no longer able to change a situation, we are challenged to change ourselves." *– Viktor Frankl, author, Nobel Laureate*

One of the greatest motivations to stick with your weight loss program is seeing the pounds drop. When you hit the dreaded "plateau" and your weight loss levels off, you might get discouraged. Maybe a weight loss plateau is the REAL reason you are dissatisfied with your Lap-Band as you have been losing and gaining the same 2 pounds for several months now, while you see your friends steadily lose with a bypass or a sleeve. This might lead you to wonder, "Is something wrong with my band?" Rather than doubt your band or yourself, take the time to understand what triggers a plateau and how to move past it. Here are a few key questions:

Are you eating enough protein? How many grams of protein a day should you eat?

Remember my First Rule of WLS Eating: Lean Protein First. But how much is enough? The most common recommendation is 50 to 60 grams of protein per day for the average person, but some bariatric programs push 80 or 90 grams of protein a day on their weight loss surgery patients. I think this is really too much. If you only have a small pouch above your band, then how can you possibly consume that much protein? I suggest that my patients comfortably eat about 45 to 55 grams of protein a day, with much of that coming from lean sources such as vegetables, whole grains, beans, tofu, and fish (see Appendix E). The exact number depends on the size of the patient. A 5-foot-tall grandmother shouldn't (and probably couldn't) eat the same amount of protein as a 6'2" college student.

"Yes, I know the number of grams, but how much should I eat?"

Turning abstract numbers into practice is a struggle in itself. As a guideline, I recommend the "1-2-3 Rule for Protein." You should eat:

1 ounce of protein for breakfast,

2 ounces for lunch, and

3 ounces for dinner.

Remember, one ounce of meat = about seven grams of protein. And how much is an ounce? A good approximation is that a deck of cards is about the size of three ounces of protein. To get two ounces, just approximate a portion size about two-thirds the size of a deck of cards. Another easy trick is to remember that one boiled egg is about one ounce of protein.

Here's an example of the 1-2-3 Rule in action:

Breakfast: Big glass of water, boiled egg, small banana = About 7 grams of protein in the egg

Lunch: Big glass of water, super-large mixed salad with raw veggies and 2 ounces of chicken = About 14 grams of protein in the chicken

Dinner: Big glass of water, veggies, 3-ounce grilled fish filet on a bed of couscous = 21 grams of protein in the fish

7+14+21 = 42 grams of protein for the day.

"But Dr. Vuong, that's not enough protein!" you shout. You would be correct if you counted only "animal" sources of protein. Veggies and whole grains like couscous also contain protein. This one-day sample meal plan easily has over 50 grams of protein, or more protein than you probably need in a day.

I also want my patients to focus on LEAN sources of protein. Getting 30 grams of protein from a protein bullet drink won't cut it. Relying on pre-formulated drinks uses the same false logic as thinking you are doing well by drinking a diet soda or selecting canned tuna. Not all sources of protein are the same. You are much better off eating beans, whole grains, tofu, and fish **most of the time** than you are drinking a protein shake **every** morning or eating a lot of meat products, like luncheon meat or beef jerky. String cheese is NOT a healthy snack, and dipping your apple slices in peanut butter (to add more protein) is NOT a good option.

Here are some bad protein choices (i.e. high in fat and sodium and low in nutrients): peanut butter, string cheese, cheese crackers, beef jerky, luncheon meat, hamburgers without the buns, refried beans, protein shots, bacon, sausage patties, meatballs, and pizza toppings.

Here are some good protein choices: fresh green smoothies, couscous, quinoa, bulgar, kale, broccoli, lentils, beans, tofu, and fish.

Could it be that you are drinking your daily calories? List any drinks you are consuming that contain calories and how frequently. What is wrong with diet drinks?

"THE MAJORITY OF THE CALORIES CONSUMED IN AMERICA NOW ARE EMPTY CALORIES FROM LIQUID DRINKS."

A Skinny Vanilla Latte Venti made with non-fat milk and no whipped cream from Starbucks still has 160 calories! I have a patient who used to drink six or seven of these a day, even after she had her weight loss surgery. She believed she was making a good choice because they're made with non-fat milk and are called "skinny," but those seven drinks still added about 1,000 calories a day to her diet! When she found out the REAL skinny on this drink, she quit her habit, and she is now well on her way to weight loss success.

What about alcohol? Are you consuming empty calories with poor alcohol choices? One margarita can pack up to 600 calories, so a three-margarita girls-night-out could add up to1800 calories in drinks alone. If you are at a party and absolutely must have a drink, wine is a lower-calorie option. I love to socialize, and by no means am I a tea-totaler, but I try to keep everything in perspective and understand my reasons for imbibing that night.

"What about all of those energy drinks, Dr. Vuong?" If you "need" them for energy, then probably you: 1) are not getting proper nutrition, so your body seeks nourishment from any quickly available source; 2) need more sleep; or 3) have fallen for the multi-billion-dollar marketing hype. Most of these drinks pack *a lot* of calories. They take you on a sugar high only to let you crash a couple of hours later. Remember that calories are our body's source of energy, so anything that calls itself "energy," even if it has a picture of someone running uphill, is going to be full of calories. The so-called "5 hour energy shots" have received a lot of televised scrutiny lately because of multiple deaths related to their consumption. The FDA investigated five deaths linked to consumption of Monster energy drinks. In one case, a 16 year-old girl died after consuming two 24-ounce Monsters in 24 hours, leading to caffeine toxicity.

"What is the problem with diet sodas?"_ Plenty. One morning in my office, three new patients were sitting at the kitchen table, waiting for my dietitian to develop a 1,200-calorie meal plan with them. I came in and poured myself a small cup of coffee and added two sugar packets. One of the patients with a BMI of almost 55, said, "Dr. Vuong, you are setting a bad example for us. You are supposed to be demonstrating healthy choices."

"What's the problem?" I asked.

She said, "Why are you putting sugar packets in your coffee? That's bad for you!"

I responded, "I know where sugar comes from—sugar cane—but I don't know where the stuff in pink, blue, or yellow packets comes from."

It's not any one item, like sugar or butter, that causes us to be obese. It's what we do most days that matters. It doesn't make sense for you to order a Big Mac, french fries, and a milkshake—these three items add up to almost

2,100 calories—and then think that you are making a good choice because you've also ordered a DIET Coke. People often over-consume diet sodas because they think they are harmless. Some studies suggest that diet soda drinkers consume more calories by the end of the day because they splurge on other foods. In addition, diet sodas have no nutritional value and a lot of chemicals. I would rather enjoy a small amount of real sugar than a lot of artificial sweeteners. Our bodies usually know how to process and handle sugar—but I'm not sure they know what to do with artificial sweeteners, especially not in the copious amounts present in the typical American diet. Other "healthy" or "harmless" additives or substitutes also contain a lot of chemicals.

The next time you are in a restaurant or at a social gathering, look around and see who is drinking diet soda. I'll bet you'll find it is mostly the overweight people. If you don't want to look like them, don't copy their habits. I'm not saying it's ok to drink regular sodas. Instead,

"STAY AWAY FROM ARTIFICIALITY AND DRINK WATER."

Could it be that you are not drinking enough water? How much water are you drinking a day? How much water should you be drinking a day?

Notice that each meal in the sample plan above starts with, "Big Glass of Water," not juice, milk, sweet tea, Gatorade, or soda.

"But Dr. V, I don't like water! How could I possibly drink that much water ?!"

"YOU ARE MOSTLY MADE OF WATER, SO THEN SAYING YOU DON'T LIKE WATER IMPLIES THAT YOU DON'T LIKE YOURSELF."

For those of you who say you don't like the "taste" of water, my answer is, you would love the "taste" of water if you were lost in the desert. You don't even need to be lost. Try this one experiment, if you don't believe me. Go for a walk or a hike where there are no convenience stores or drive-thru's around and bring only a bottle of water. Leave it at the starting point, work up a sweat, and when you get back to the start, just try NOT to drink that water! You won't be able to; it will look too tempting. Do this exercise a couple of times and you'll be hooked on the "taste" of water. Why do I put "taste" in quotation marks? **Because water has no taste**. If your water has a taste, it is not pure water, and you might try filtering it. More likely you dislike the *lack* of artificial taste to which you've become accustomed in your drinks.

How much water you should drink depends on your size and activity level, but it is usually around eight to ten eight-ounce glasses per day. I drink 10 glasses of water a day, and I weigh 135 pounds. Put simply, drink water whenever you are thirsty to ensure you are drinking enough. Start replacing one of your non-water drinks per day with water, and every week replace another until all of your drinks are water. Of course, there will be some exceptions, but drinking water should be the main way you quench your thirst.

"I heard you can drink too much water! Is this true, Dr. Vuong?"

There is one psychological illness that drives people to drink excessive amounts of water. They will drink it from anywhere—directly from the tap, toilet water, doggie bowls, sewer drainage pipes, anywhere. So, unless you are drinking water from the rain gutters at your house, you should be able to have that next bottle. Some people also drink too much water when they are training for a grueling athletic endeavor, such as a marathon, that makes them overly nervous about dehydration. This is extremely rare, as it requires drinking many cups of water every mile or so, which would make most people sick.

On average the human body is about 60%-65% water—men have a slightly higher percentage than women because they typically have more lean muscle. Muscle contains a much larger percentage of water (75%) than does fat (10%). Your blood is 83% water.

Consider this: **your brain is 75% water.** We lose water all of the time. We urinate it out, we sweat it out, we snore it out. Humans need to replace about 2.4 liters of water a day. But we don't replace the loss with water. We replace it with soda, tea, coffee, energy drinks—and then we wonder why we get headaches. We wonder why we can't focus, do the math, shake the blues, get off the couch on Sunday, or remember where we parked the car. It's not a matter of depression, will power, or senility. It's a matter of dehydration. If you are not drinking enough water, then you are dehydrating your brain, *starving* it. And your brain controls everything!

Without enough water, you will have headaches and feel sluggish and dizzy. If you replace water with sugary drinks or add a lot of chemicals, you will feel jittery and then crash. Drinking water steadily will keep your brain and body fueled and feeling good.

You will never have the life you want if you don't drink enough water. Because we lose water all of the time, and our brain is water, and our brain controls everything, you'll never have the career you want, marriage you desire, patience for your child, or inspiration for your book if you don't drink enough water. So...

"YOU NEED TO SUPERHYDRATE."

Could it be that you are not eating enough? How many times a day should you eat after weight loss surgery?

Our clinic teaches patients to eat three meals a day, plus a snack if they are diabetic or are truly hungry between meals. If you are hungry between meals, do not "tough it out" until the next mealtime. This is because after your surgery, you physically can't eat enough at one sitting to make up for that hunger craving, leaving you frustrated. Help your hunger by drinking a glass of water. I had a patient who used to work all day, skip meals, and be ravenous when she got home; then she would eat a large easy meal, like spaghetti. She couldn't understand why she wasn't losing weight, when it was clear that she was making poor choices. Don't fall into that cycle. Have the snack, and your next meal will be an appropriately-sized, WLS meal. Of course, by snack, I mean a good snack—not candy, cookies, chips, cheese crackers, or anything else that can cause your blood sugar to spike and crash. **This is not a free pass to splurge.** Have the rest of your breakfast banana, a handful of blueberries, or jicama sticks, for example.

Unlike some clinics, we teach our patients that breakfast is NOT the most important meal of the day, but we do encourage them to eat something in the morning. Patients need to think about breakfast in a different way from what Denny's Restaurant would like. A banana with two big glasses of water is a perfect breakfast. I also suggest fresh green smoothies made with an emulsifier (like Nutribullet, NutriNinja, or Vitamix), containing fruit and some leafy greens such as spinach or kale. Protein powders are optional. I drink a fresh green smoothie most mornings.

You don't need to eat bacon, eggs, cereal, oatmeal, or yogurt to be healthy.

Q: Who in America eats yogurt every morning, trying to lose weight and be healthy?

A: Fat people!

If you don't want to be one of them, don't do what they do!

Change your idea of breakfast. I often eat freshly plucked spinach or kale leaves as I am thinning out my garden in the mornings. Sometimes I grab a handful of chocolate cherry tomatoes from the vine by the kitchen door as I head to work. My daughter enjoys peaches or red bell peppers for breakfast as much as she does a mango or a banana. Breakfast foods don't need to be different from other foods. In fact, 15 minutes of light exercise in the morning, like stretching, jumping jacks, push-ups, yoga, or meditation is probably more beneficial to our health than the typical American breakfast of cereal, bagels, sausage biscuits, donuts, or pancakes.

In my book, *Ultimate Gastric Sleeve Success*, I introduced Kizzie's Rule, named after my daughter: **You can eat all the fresh fruits and vegetables you want, as much as you want, anytime you want.** Incorporate this rule when planning your meals by focusing on the fruits and vegetables. You're also after a **variety** of fruits and vegetables. Practice this rule during snacks, as well. Eventually, eliminate snacks altogether, because in order to lose weight, you have to reduce your caloric intake, which means you must let yourself get hungry. Don't be a GRAZER!

"SNACKING NEEDS TO HAVE A LIMITED ROLE IN YOUR LIFE."

What is the minimum number of calories you should consume to avoid metabolic slowdown? How can you combat a slow metabolism?

Any very low caloric diet (VLCD) requires monitoring by a physician. These are typically meal replacement diets of less than 1,000 calories per day (such as is the Optifast 800 Meal Replacement Program). The physician should perform regular, routine lab work to check your blood chemistries and your kidney and liver functions.

The medical field believes that when caloric intake drops to below 1,000 calories per day, human metabolism will slow down. This is a natural, evolutionary response. Think back to the caveman. When humans had to scavenge for food that was not always readily available, our bodies became very efficient at storing energy in the form of fat, which would tide us through times when we might not be able to eat much for a few days. When food became scarce, our metabolism would slow down in order to conserve energy, at least until food became plentiful again. Since gastric band surgery will take you close to the 1,000-calorie threshold (my patients eat 1,100-1,200 calories a day), your body will want to go into hibernation mode. Your job is to keep this from happening. How do you do this?

With two simple steps as follows.

Step 1: Make sure you are getting the best nutrition you can.

This means eating real food, avoiding empty calories, preparing fresh meals, and buying organic foods whenever possible. This will give your body all of the micronutrients and building blocks it needs to perform its normal daily chemical reactions that keep you feeling good.

You can accomplish this by following my second rule:

"FILL YOUR POUCH WITH THE MOST NUTRITIOUS FOOD YOU CAN MOST OF THE TIME."

Step 2: Exercise regularly.

This will keep your metabolism going by releasing natural hormones that control your "fight or flight" response. Have you heard of a "runner's high?" Sometimes, getting started with an exercise routine is tough, but think back about how great you felt after a workout—in addition to the pride of accomplishment, you probably also felt energized and alert. That's a natural response. It had very little to do with your new gym equipment, your personal trainer with rock hard abs, or your perfectly set iTunes playlist. It had everything to do with what a wonderful machine the human body is. If you are significantly overweight, you can get started with any activity you like that makes you **break one bead of sweat**, and you can call it exercise. If you are further along in your weight loss but have stalled with just a few pounds left to your goal, then you will need to step up your exercise to break the plateau—and by "step up" I mean varying your activity as well as increasing your intensity. Exercise needs to be pleasurable and not feel like "work" or a "chore." It needs to become a part of your personal identity, much like healthy food choices do, and not something you hope to incorporate on occasion.

EXERCISE = ANY PHYSICAL ACTIVITY YOU LIKE THAT CAUSES YOU TO BREAK ONE BEAD OF SWEAT

If you are significantly overweight or just getting started in your journey, exercise could be as simple as putting on your pants, cleaning your house, or washing your car. If you've lost a lot of pounds or are near your goal weight, then these lower-level activities will no longer be exercise because they will no longer be strenuous enough to make you sweat. Switch to walking around the block, and when that becomes too easy, run. Instead of trekking through the park, go hiking. Instead of light water aerobics, swim laps. As you get thinner and fitter, increase your level of physical activity continually.

Have you ever heard, "The last 20 pounds are the hardest to lose?" My guess is that people who complain about this would benefit from following the steps outlined above. The last 20 pounds are really the same as the first 20, but your body percentages are different (assuming the pounds are not comprised of excess skin, which needs to be surgically removed. Do not be afraid to look into skin removal surgery.) The choices that allowed you to lose the first 50 percent of your excess weight will not be good enough to help you lose the last 50 percent. If you lost 50 pounds by skipping the chips with your daily sandwich, then to lose the next 50 pounds, you will need to keep skipping the chips, but also replace the sandwich with a salad. If you lost 80 pounds by incorporating small bouts of exercise into your day, like taking the stairs, then in order for you to lose the next 80 pounds, you can't rest between floors. You've got to run up those stairs! Try fresh veggies, tofu, lentils, and fish. Lace up the running shoes and go pound some pavement! Don't worry, you don't have to do all of these things at once, but do more of them the leaner and healthier you become.

Keep making the healthiest choices possible all along the way, and everything will work itself out. In fact, if you are doing well with your weight loss, then you probably need to throw out the scale. Only *you* will know what "doing well" means...

"YOU HAVE PROGRESSED BEYOND WHAT THE SCALE CAN TELL YOU ABOUT YOUR HEALTH, MUCH LESS YOUR JOURNEY."

The scale at this point does not tell you how far you've come, how great you feel, how much more intimate your marriage is, how good each morning feels.

Are you consuming empty calories (calories without any nutritious value)? Any at all? Write down everything you have eaten since breakfast yesterday morning and evaluate your choices.

If you are losing neither weight nor inches, and especially if you are GAINING weight, then you are consuming too many extra calories—pure and simple, right? That's probably what most "experts" would tell you, but it's not necessarily the case. Perhaps your quality of nutrition rather than your quantity of calories is the problem. Are you still eating string cheese or beef jerky for protein? Are you still having peanut butter crackers for an afternoon snack? Do you still start every morning with a protein shake?

"FOCUS LESS ON 'CALORIES IN' AND MORE ON 'NUTRITION IN'."

We focus too much on calories consumed. I think this is a product of years of dieting and "health" marketing gimmicks. **The key to good health lies in nutrition, not calories.** Nutrition is found in fresh fruits and vegetables, not very much in meat, and definitely not in human-made products. The most nutritious foods with the fewest calories are leafy greens, such as salad leaves, kale, arugula, and spinach. These are foods that you need to be able to eat with your band. If you can't, then you are probably too tight. If you have a revisional surgery, these are the foods you will need to eat.

Keeping a food diary is essential to long-term weight loss. There are no excuses when you keep a food diary—the evidence is right there in front of you. Our minds work to avoid hurting us psychologically and allow us to forget things, which can sometimes undermine our weight-loss efforts. Remember that time you were going to eat just one Girl Scout cookie, and before you knew it, the whole box was gone? If you know that you will be accountable for every cookie, it's not as easy to keep eating. When you know that you will have to count up all the empty slots in that cookie box and calculate how many calories the missing cookies contained and write it all in your food diary, you'll find yourself able to stop after one or two, or maybe you won't even open the box at all. **But at some point you will need to ask, "How did these cookies even get into my house?"**

People who have lasting weight loss often keep food diaries. They are dedicated to writing down not only the calories they consume, but also the activities they do, and all of the emotions they were feeling while eating or exercising. Some people prefer to use a paper notebook, but there are also lots of websites with resources and references to help you log everything. Mobile apps will even allow you to log your food intake on the spot! We like MyFitnessPal in my clinic, but any convenient app will work. You could even just take a photo of everything you eat—if you choose to do this, then place something in the picture, like a quarter or fork, to help the dietitian gauge (pro)portion sizes.

One time, I saw a television news story about a woman who had lost 150 pounds without surgery. Her strategy was simply to pack all of her food for the day into a small box. She could not eat anything unless it came out of that box, except for water. While this sounds extreme, it was very effective. But when I stop and think about it, that "food box" was basically the equivalent of her food diary.

Instead of writing down what she ate after the fact, she preemptively logged her intake by packing her entire day's worth of food into a small box.

Keeping a food journal is like anything else—it's a little difficult to get started, but once you get going it becomes second nature. Saying goodbye to those pounds forever is worth that extra bit of effort, especially if you are considering a revisional bariatric surgery, which is much more complicated and riskier than the original surgery. Make sure that you've exhausted all nonsurgical options prior to "going under the knife" again.

Summary and Tips: "There is no such thing as a Weight Loss Plateau."

1) Write down ALL of the protein sources you consume. Be specific.

____

____

____

____

Now go back and circle the lean sources from your list. Use Appendix E as a reference. Eliminate all non-lean sources of protein from your diet.

2) Write down all of the liquids you consume.

____

____

____

____

Of those listed, circle the ones you will stop drinking.

3) Your BRAIN IS WATER, and it controls EVERYTHING. Write down how much water you drink everyday. ____________________.

If that amount is less than 100 oz or 10 bottles, then write down how much you will increase it to. ____________________

4) Focus more on NUTRITION and less on CALORIES. Search for a book on nutrition (not a diet book) and commit to reading it. Write down the title here.

5) The scale is just a number. It does not say anything about you as a person. Pretend you are interviewing for your dream job and you have to describe yourself. Write down 5 great qualities that best describe you!

4

A Finicky Band and Other Things That Impede Weight Loss Success

"Success is not final. Failure is not fatal. It is the courage to continue that counts." *– Winston Churchill, English Prime Minister*

You were probably careful to avoid the traps and dangers that could derail you when you first started your weight loss journey. You cut out all sodas, even diet, because you didn't want to stretch out your pouch. ALL of the junk was cleared out of your house and removed from secret hiding places. You shared a meal with your spouse when ordering, and that was even after you had made sure not to graze during the day. You stopped using straws and maybe even ate with a baby spoon for awhile. Then life happened. Maybe a few of those old bad habits came back, and maybe you've worked hard on getting rid of them again. But even if you are doing everything right, you still might not be successful with your band and wonder why.

Mushy Food Syndrome—I discuss Mushy Food Syndrome in detail in *Ultimate Gastric Sleeve Success*, but I will summarize it here. Mushy foods are also called "slider foods," because they tend to "go down easily." A lot of weight loss surgery patients, especially banded patients, think this is a good thing, but it is not. Mushy foods are typically high in calories, but low in nutrition. I STRONGLY advise that you do not get hooked on eating mushy foods, like mashed potatoes, refried beans, yogurt, pretzels, peanut butter, and pudding. Here's why:

Question: What is your WEIGHT going to do if you eat mostly foods that are high in calories and low in nutrition?

***Answer:** Plateau or increase*

Question: What is your ENERGY LEVEL going to be if you eat mostly foods that are high in calories and low in nutrition?

***Answer:** Low and sluggish*

Question: What is your ATTITUDE going to be if you eat mostly foods that are high in calories and low in nutrition?

***Answer:** Grumpy, moody, not very pleasant! Why? Because, "Dr. Vuong, I'm barely eating, I have no energy, and gosh darn it, I'm not even losing any weight!"*

This cycle of poor choices/poor results is what I call the "Mushy Food Syndrome." If this seems to describe your situation, then chances are your Band is too tight. You should see your surgeon for a deflation.

"IF YOU ARE ABLE TO EAT ONLY MUSHY FOODS, YOU NEED A DEFLATION, NOT MORE FLUID, EVEN IF YOU ARE GAINING WEIGHT!"

You need to be deflated so that you can eat Super Foods, which are the opposite of Mushy Foods. Super foods are relatively *high in nutrition* but *low in calories* (can you name a few?). Eating Super Foods is key to success with *any* weight loss surgery.

Most of the foods overweight people eat would fit into the category of Mushy Foods, including chips, bread, tortillas, mashed potatoes, applesauce, yogurt, pretzels, cake, candy bars, fast food, fries, pizza, and processed foods, to name a few. These "food" items make up the vast majority of the meals for many Americans, yet they fail to nourish our bodies. Remember this:

"EVERY MEAL IS AN OPPORTUNITY TO NOURISH YOUR BODY."

So eat Super Foods to nourish your body and don't slip into Mushy Food Syndrome.

Sweet tooth. When my daughter Kizzie was 6 years old, she lost her first tooth. One day Kizzie asked her mother, "Mommy, what if it was my sweet tooth that I lost?! Will I get another sweet tooth?" I don't know where Kizzie got the idea, but she heard the phrase somewhere and thought that she had an actual tooth that allowed her to enjoy sweets. The idea of the sweet tooth starts at a very young age.

Gastric bypass patients can get a side effect called dumping syndrome. Dumping occurs when a bypass patient eats something too high in sugar (candy, ice cream, juice, etc...), and it causes nausea, cramps, and explosive diarrhea. This will deter patients from eating sweets most of the time. But while some patients (and some surgeons) think that gastric bypass surgery will stop the sweet tooth permanently, it doesn't. Here is why:

- Not every bypass patient gets dumping syndrome after surgery, and
- Most bypass patients will eventually lose dumping syndrome.

The drive for sweets can be powerful.

Amanda's Story

Amanda had done well with her gastric bypass, performed through a different program 4 years earlier, but had regained about 50 pounds. She came to see me for help. I asked her to describe her dumping to me.

She said, "It's terrible. I get awful tummy pains, nausea, vomiting, and diarrhea. I'm curled up on the floor in a fetal position, rolling around for a couple of hours!"

I asked her why she thought she was regaining weight, and I will never forget her answer.

She said, "I can't stop eating sweets."

I replied, "But I thought you said you had terrible dumping?"

"Yes, I do…" and with a panicked look in her eyes, she said, "That's crazy isn't it Dr. V? I REALLY NEED YOUR HELP!"

****

That's when it dawned on me **how much more powerful our minds are than our bodies.** This patient was willing to put her body through pain and suffering, but not address her psychological need for sweets.

Lap-Band patients cannot rely on dumping to fight sugar cravings, so this could be a major culprit of your weight regain. As you can see from the example above, the mind is where the answer lies. Reevaluate your food choices, and see if you are sneaking in more sweets than you realize. For example, I consider peanut butter (including peanut butter crackers) a sweet. A few other "sweets" might include sweet tea (even if you use artificial sweeteners), diet sodas, small candy bars, most breakfast cereals, pastries, pancakes, waffles, or fancy coffee drinks. Fresh fruit doesn't count because a lot of nutrition goes with its natural sugars, but otherwise sweets are just empty calories that waste room in your pouch and sidetrack you from your weight loss goals.

"I can't seem to get back to the 'sweet spot'." Many Lap-Band patients will be disappointed to read this:

"I BELIEVE THE GREEN ZONE SWEET SPOT IS A LAP-BAND MYTH."

Most Lap-Band surgeons will disagree with my statement and suggest I can't find the green zone because I do not provide enough patient aftercare. In fact, I provide a tremendous amount of aftercare (as well as pre-care), and my band patients have above average weight loss. But even with all of the education I provide patients, a high percentage slip in and out of the "sweet spot." Eventually, I decided that the "sweet spot" is a myth because as time passes with your band, your anatomy changes, and the "sweet spot" moves. After all, there are only a finite number of adjustments, and as you lose weight, the fat around your stomach changes. I think at some point adding fluid to the band only *obstructs* you and no longer *restricts* you. Why does this happen? Maybe it's due to scar tissue around the band. Maybe the esophagus dilated and is now a reservoir for food. We are not sure. The healthcare industry does not know everything about how the gastric band works.

I have performed enough endoscopic studies now to know that most banded patients don't really have a "pouch" above the band, so most food sits in the esophagus. An esophagus is intended to be a passage for food to travel from your mouth to your stomach. The esophagus works both dependently and independently from your conscious control to keep itself clear of any food or saliva. In other words, 1) you can consciously swallow, which causes your esophagus to push food down or 2) your esophagus can independently sense food or saliva and squeeze on its own. This squeezing process is called peristalsis. Much of the "fullness" or "pressure" a patient feels with the band initially could well be pain caused by food sitting in the esophagus, not from a full pouch above the band. Since your esophagus is not intended to hold the food sitting in it above the band, it will inevitably dilate. I think this esophageal dilation leads to esophageal spasm and inappropriate functioning of the gastric band.

As your esophagus dilates and spasms, its diameter begins to expand, making it difficult to get back into that Green Zone. As the esophagus expands, it can hold more food without causing discomfort, making you think the food has "gone down" even though your band is very tight. I see this often on barium swallows: a patient comes in complaining of weight gain and being able to "eat anything" and asks for a fill. When I do a barium swallow and ask her if the she thinks the barium has gone down, she says "Yes." Then I show her the image on the screen, which shows all of the barium is still sitting in her esophagus. I ask, "If this liquid barium is sticking in your esophagus, then where do you think the hamburger is sitting?" At this point, the realization sets in, especially when she sees her esophagus spastically squeezing to push the barium through.

If your band has slipped and been deflated, it's even harder to get back to the sweet spot. As the amount of fluid returns close to the level at which the slip occurred, the band, more often than not, will reslip, and you have to be deflated again. Does this sound familiar?

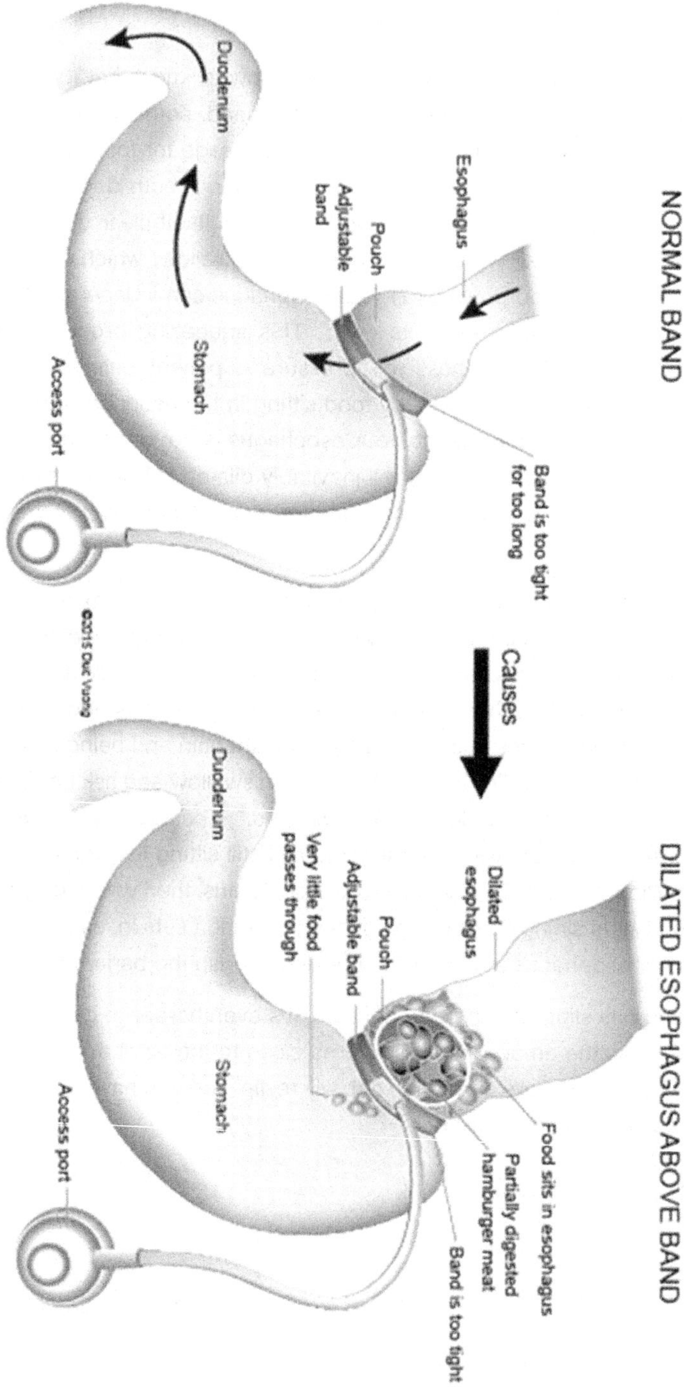
NORMAL BAND
Esophagus
Pouch
Adjustable band
Band is too tight for too long
Duodenum
Stomach
Access port
Causes
DILATED ESOPHAGUS ABOVE BAND
Dilated esophagus
Pouch
Adjustable band
Very little food passes through
Food sits in esophagus
Partially digested hamburger meat
Band is too tight
Duodenum
Stomach
Access port
©2015 Duc Vuong

A little fluid out, a little fluid in. This dilated esophagus/tight band cycle is vicious: a little fluid out and patients feel no restriction, but a little fluid in and she becomes completely obstructed. "One day I can eat anything. The next day, everything gets stuck." Patients often refer to this as "a finicky band." This can be very frustrating not only for patients but also for surgeons. I suspect the cycle stems from a dilated esophagus that allows food to sit too long and a band that is too tight. In addition, over time a pseudocapsule or "scar tissue" might build up underneath the band and around the stomach, causing unintentional restriction and possibly obstruction when a little fluid is added.

At some point, the cycle needs to be broken. As a preventative measure to the development of a "finicky" band, I place my patients on what I call "Lap-Band Vacations." During a Lap-Band Vacation, I deflate their bands, put them on liquids for two weeks, and perform an EGD. I'm unaware of any data that this will help, but for me, it makes sense to give your esophagus a break from the band, just like you need a vacation from your job.

Sometimes, the esophagus might be so dilated, spastic, or "corkscrewed" that it requires deflation for several months before returning to normal, if it ever does. In severe cases, your surgeon might advise semi-emergent band removal. I've seen one band patient whose esophagus had become so spastic that it was shaped like the letter "c" instead of a straight tube. Check with your surgeon to see what he recommends.

Bariatric surgeons now agree that in order to be successful with the band, a patient must be diligent with follow-up care. The band is a mechanical device and, like your car, it needs regular maintenance. But sometimes, even when the patient does everything she is supposed to do, the band can still have problems.

Summary and Tips: "Am I impeding my own SUCCESS?"

1) Mushy Food Syndrome. Write down all of the soft slider foods you are eating.

2) Sweet Tooth. Write down any sweets that you eat. Don't forget to include pastries, cereal, candy, and sodas.

3) Every meal is an opportunity to nourish your body. Write down one new nutritious food you will add to your diet, like salad everyday for lunch, water with every meal, or fruit as a snack.

4) How often are you getting stuck or regurgitating food? Write down every episode for this past week/month/few months, including what got stuck and the occasion.

5) Our minds are much more powerful than our bodies. Close your eyes every morning and visualize yourself as thin and healthy. Do this 10 times during the day.

5

Basic Anatomy and Technical Terms

"To acquire knowledge, one must study; but to acquire wisdom, one must observe." *– Marilyn vos Savant*

Before we proceed any further, we need to review some basic anatomy to lay the groundwork for discussions about revisional surgery options. It will also help you understand visually why you are feeling some of the symptoms you have with the band. Bookmark this page as you may want to refer back to it, especially when we start discussing some of the surgical revision options. I also recommend you purchase a used basic anatomy book such as *Atlas of Human Anatomy* by Dr. Frank Netter for reference.

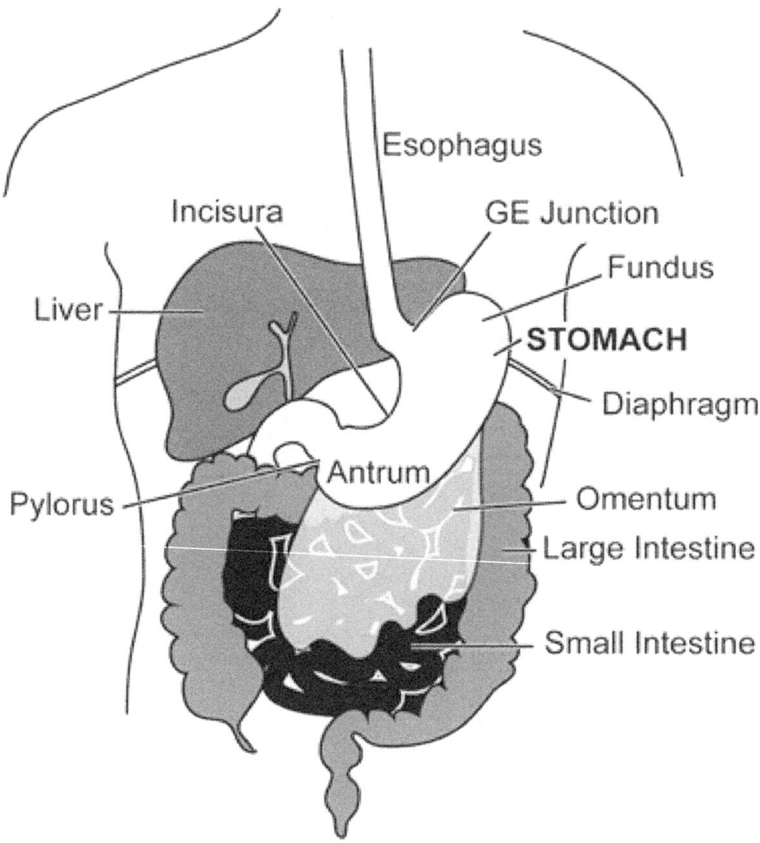

This is a diagram of a normal stomach. Note these anatomic areas:

GE Junction: This stands for the gastroesophageal junction (GEJ), where the esophagus becomes the stomach.

Crus (or "crura" in plural form) of the diaphragm: Your diaphragm is the sheet of muscle that separates your chest (thoracic) cavity from your abdominal cavity. It is a thin muscle, but as it progresses toward the middle of your body, it thickens into two more pronounced muscular pillars called the crura. Like a Roman cathedral, there is one pillar for each side of the body. The opening (hiatus) between the left and right crura is the space where the esophagus, aorta, nerves, and a few other structures extend from your chest into your abdomen.

Hiatus: The opening defined by the left and right crura of the diaphragm. When the hiatus is larger than normal, parts of your stomach can slide up into your chest cavity. This is known as a hiatal hernia.

Fundus: The top portion of your stomach. It has the potential to stretch.

Omentum: The protective sheet of fat that lies over your intestines. We are learning more about it every day. We used to think all the omentum did was "shield" our abdominal organs from harm, but now we think that it is an endocrine organ—in other words, it reacts to chemical signals to affect biological change in our bodies. The omentum becomes quite fatty with obesity, and scientists now believe this is one of the major causes of comorbidities. The extra weight of the fatty omentum exerts pressure on the blood vessels and organs, making them have to work harder to keep our bodies functioning properly.

Greater Curve: The long curve in your stomach. It is attached to your omentum and lies near the colon.

Lesser Curve: The shorter curve in your stomach. It is thicker and less stretchy than the greater curve.

Incisura: The bend of your lesser curve.

Antrum: The area of the stomach right before your pylorus. It performs a "churning" action that mixes food with stomach juices to speed up digestion.

Pylorus: The muscle at the bottom outlet of your stomach that controls the rate at which partially digested food leaves your stomach and goes into your duodenum.

Mesentery: This is the fan-shaped suspensory ligament of the jejunum and ileum. The mesentery contains the blood vessels, nerves, and lymphatic channels of the small bowel. In obesity, the mesentery, like the greater omentum, can enlarge with additional quantities of fat, thereby making weight loss surgery more difficult. This is especially challenging in intestinal rerouting surgeries such as the gastric bypass and duodenal switch.

Duodenum: The first portion of your small intestine that is responsible for a variety of digestive processes. It absorbs most of the nutrients and calories.

Jejunum: The second portion of your small intestine. It is usually the point where the bowel is transected (divided) during a gastric bypass.

Ileum: The third portion of the small intestine that connects to the colon. The ileum is transected during a duodenal switch surgery and connected to the duodenum.

Technical Terms

Medical terminology is its own language. Below are some common terms that you might encounter when reading this book or discussing your options with your surgeon. You may want to refer back to this section frequently, so bookmark it for easy reference.

Adhesions: When communicating with patients, surgeons often refer to adhesions as "scar tissue," which is partially but not entirely accurate. Adhesions are fibrous bands that form between two membranous surfaces, such as internal organs and tissues, as a result of the body's natural healing process from surgery. They can be "filmy" and easy to take down, or "thick" and possibly necessitate a difficult dissection to separate the two tissues without causing injury to either one. Because adhesions form at different rates and varying intensities with each individual, surgeons will not know the extent of adhesions until the time of surgery. This adds an element of unpredictability for both the surgeon and the patient.

Anastomosis: An anastomosis is the surgical connection between two separate tubular organs, which in this case involves the gastrointestinal system.

- ***Gastrojejunal Anastomosis:*** The surgical connection between the stomach and the jejunum, usually seen in the gastric bypass and minigastric bypass.
- ***Jejenojejunal Anastomosis:*** The surgical connection between two separate sections of jejunum as seen in the gastric bypass.
- ***Dudenoileal Anastomosis:*** The surgical connection formed from the duodenum to the ileum as seen in the duodenal switch.
- ***End-to-End Anastomosis:*** A method of surgical connection in which the ends of each tube are reattached, like connecting a garden hose to a spigot. In the case of a bypass, the new small stomach pouch can be connected to the end of the jejunum.

- ***End-to-Side Anastomosis:*** A method of surgical connection in which the end of one tube (in the case of a bypass, the new small stomach pouch) is connected to the side of another tube (in the case of a bypass, the side of the jejunum, as opposed to the end.)

Alimentary Limb: This is the segment of small intestine down which food travels after a gastric bypass or duodenal switch. It is the far (distal) end of the intestine that was transected and brought up to connect to the new pouch. In the case of a gastric bypass, the distal jejunum connects to the new smaller stomach pouch. For the duodenal switch, the distal ileum is brought up and connected to the duodenum.

Roux Limb: This is another name for the alimentary limb of a gastric bypass, named after the Swedish surgeon Cesar Roux, who is credited with inventing the gastric bypass procedure for weight loss.

Biliopancreatic Limb: This is the segment of small intestine down which the stomach juices, bile, and liver secretions travel to meet up with the food in the alimentary limb.

Open Surgery: Open surgery is the “traditional” approach to surgery in which a large incision is made along the midline of the abdomen. The surgeon splits muscle fibers in the middle of the belly to give access to the organs. The length of the incision is dependent on the nature of the case and the experience of the surgeon.

Laparoscopic Surgery: Starting in the 1980’s and gaining momentum in the 1990’s, laparoscopy revolutionized the field of surgery. The surgeon, instead of making one large incision, makes a few small incisions and inflates the abdominal cavity with carbon dioxide gas. The inflated belly is called a pneumoperitoneum. The process creates space for the surgeon to introduce a fiberoptic camera and long surgical instruments into the abdomen. This approach results in less pain and a faster recovery time for patients. With the recent improvement in camera optics and advancements in instrumentation, many technically difficult surgeries can now be performed laparoscopically.

Malabsorption: This is the reduced, incomplete, or altered uptake (absorption) of ingested substances, such as food, nutrients, and medicines. Malabsorption is more common in surgeries where the intestines are rerouted, such as the Roux-N-Y gastric bypass, minigastric bypass, and duodenal switch, because the part of the small intestine (the duodenum and much of the jejunum) that is responsible for the absorption of those substances is bypassed.

Staple line: The surgeon uses a special instrument, often called a "staple gun" or "stapler," to divide tissue. The stapler clamps down on the tissue and fires 6 rows of staples. Then a knife blade cuts in between the third and fourth rows, leaving three rows on each side of the divided tissue. This accomplishes two purposes: 1) to seal the tissues and 2) to separate the tissues. In the case of a sleeve gastrectomy, the sleeve will have three rows of staples to help seal it, and the specimen (the side of the stomach to be removed) will be sealed with three rows of staples so as to not release stomach juices during extraction. Older staplers used to staple off but not cut, so surgeons had to manually cut in between the staples. In revisional surgery, tissues can be thicker due to adhesions and fibrosis, so the staples often have to be longer. The risk of staple line failure, leading to a leak, is therefore greater in revisions.

Staple line reinforcement versus Oversewing: Some surgeons use buttressing material to reinforce the staple line. Think of this dissolvable material as a liner over the staples that helps control bleeding and possibly decreases leaks, but adds cost to the case. Some surgeons choose to run a stitch over the staple line (this is called "oversewing"), which cuts down on the surgery's cost and has acceptable results. I use buttressing material and place clips along the staple line, but every surgeon is different and very little data are available to suggest a statistically significant difference between the benefits of reinforcement and those of oversewing.

Staged surgery: A staged surgery is planned as two separate surgeries—the first surgery removes the band, and the second, which usually takes place 3-6 months later, revises to a different surgery. German surgeons almost always perform revisions in two stages, as do some American surgeons. I try to do revisions in one surgery but am not always able to do so due to adhesions.

Percentage Weight Loss (%WL) versus Percentage Excess Weight Loss (%EWL): Medical doctors usually measure weight loss in terms of total body weight loss, or %WL. In other words, if you weigh 300 pounds and lose 30 pounds, you've lost 10% of your total body weight. This metric is useful because it recognizes that heavier patients tend to lose more pounds initially. On the other hand, surgeons tend to refer to percentage excess weight loss (%EWL). This is based on the weight a patient needs to be in order to have a normal BMI of 25 or less. So if you weigh 300 pounds but would need to weigh a maximum of 200 pounds to have a BMI of 25, you are 100 pounds overweight. If you lose 30 pounds, then, you have lost 30% of your excess weight. The advantage of referring to %EWL is that it sets weight loss in reference to a defined goal, i.e. a normal BMI. Surgeons typically define a %EWL of less than 50% as a "surgical failure;" however, we are starting to consider such results less as "failures" and more as "inadequate treatments."

6

Things to See Your Surgeon for ASAP

"All time is all time. It does not change. It does not lend itself to warnings or explanations. It simply is." *– Kurt Vonnegut, author*

I'm surprised by how regularly I see a band patient who has struggled for a long time before deciding to seek medical advice. Sometimes she has had abdominal pain for 6 months. Sometimes she has been sticking daily for a year. Sometimes she has had multiple "normal" studies done by her primary care doctor, who does not have any real expertise in gastric band surgery. If you are experiencing any of the symptoms below, please contact a bariatric surgeon. I can't emphasize this enough: the symptoms below indicate you need to be evaluated by an experienced bariatric surgeon, even if it means driving for hours or flying out of state.

Morning mucous production—This is a pretty common complaint from bandsters. This could be a result of seasonal allergies or just excessive mucous production from your esophagus as it tries to clear food down. Many patients explain, "I'm tight in the morning, but it seems to go away as the day goes along..." Does this sound familiar? Sometimes this morning tightness is helped by a little hot tea. If this situation becomes persistent or turns into "foaming," especially if it is accompanied by nighttime cough or reflux, then you need to see your bariatric surgeon. Your band has become too tight.

Reflux/Heartburn—One of the earliest symptoms of a tight band is reflux or heartburn. Patients often tell me that they have been experiencing increasing heartburn over several months and just ignored it because it went away when they took an antacid. But a well-adjusted band should stop acid reflux, not cause it. I'll repeat that again:

"A WELL-ADJUSTED LAP-BAND SHOULD STOP REFLUX, NOT CAUSE IT."

As acid irritation inflames the esophageal or gastric pouch tissues, the swelling of those tissues makes the opening through the band shrink. This causes the band to feel "tighter." This inflammatory cycle can lead to a lot of problems, including difficulty swallowing, or what doctors call dysphagia. If you are starting to experience reflux, call your surgeon for a check up because reflux can lead to the next two conditions.

Nighttime Cough—A nighttime cough indicates that gastric contents are refluxing upwards and irritating your airway. This suddenly wakes you up because acid fluid should not be in your lungs! Your body's natural defense against this is to cough vigorously, much like when you accidentally swallow water "the wrong way." When you are asleep and unable to protect your airway from the liquid contents in your esophagus, the liquid goes into your airway and causes you to cough. You might also wake up with a strange taste in your mouth. Some doctors call it a "brashy" taste. This is also a problem. Nighttime cough is serious enough, and it is also a precursor for even more serious problems, especially if it occurs more and more frequently.

"DO NOT IGNORE NIGHTTIME COUGH"

Worsening asthma or recurrent pneumonia—With ongoing reflux, you might aspirate (inhale) enough liquid into your lungs to exacerbate your asthma or develop recurrent pneumonia. Recurrent pneumonia in a Lap-Band patient means that the band is too tight. You should see your surgeon to get your band deflated right away.

Unfortunately, I've heard many stories of patients being admitted to the hospital for a third or fourth episode of pneumonia before the bariatric surgeon is consulted. Not every primary care doctor or hospitalist understands the connection between a band that is too tight and recurrent pneumonia. Sometimes the patient is the one who must inform the doctor of this connection!

"RECURRENT PNEUMONIA IN A BANDED PATIENT MEANS THE BAND NEEDS TO BE DEFLATED."

You can't always depend on your admitting physician to know this, so you might need to remind him that you have a Lap-Band that could be too tight. If no bariatric surgeon is available, you can always refer him to this book.

Food sticks more frequently—Does it seem like you're getting up from the table and excusing yourself to visit the bathroom more and more often to vomit up partially undigested food? At first a rare occasion, it became a weekly occurrence, and now happens daily? This is not "just a normal routine of having the band," and you should not continue to live this way. Your band is probably too tight or perhaps has slipped. **It will not get better on its own, nor will it get better if you start "following the rules" again.** The inflammatory cycle I described before has progressed too far at this point. Your band needs to be evaluated by an experienced bariatric surgeon with a barium swallow. **Prepare yourself for a possible deflation**. I have seen many patients with this problem who had surgery elsewhere and come to my clinic expecting an adjustment to be tighter.

"I can eat anything I want one day, but everything gets stuck the next day"—Have you ever seemed to have no restriction one day and are surprised you can eat a hamburger (*why are you even eating a hamburger?*) but the next day, you have trouble getting down a protein shake? Or one day, you can eat a certain food item, like shrimp, but for some reason the next day it gets stuck? Many bandsters blame this on their "finicky band," but this probably is the result of a spastic esophagus tired from trying to push food past a band that has been too tight for too long. Your esophagus works independently to clear your throat of foreign bodies, such as yesterday's chicken nuggets, meaning it can get tired. Your tired esophagus is like old spark plugs that sometimes have enough juice to start your car and sometimes don't. And every time you try to start your car, the spark plugs get weaker and weaker. Over time your esophagus might lack the "juice" to push food through your tight band. Like taking your car to a good mechanic, you need to take your band to an experienced bariatric surgeon.

Vomiting contents from more than a few hours ago—Vomiting old food is not only unpleasant, it demonstrates food stasis in your esophagus. In other words, the food you ate for lunch didn't actually pass through your band but stayed in your esophagus above your band. After a period of time, a simple burp or hiccup could bring the undigested food back up. Not only is this socially embarrassing, it shows that your band is too tight and is causing damage to your esophagus. This symptom means that your esophagus is essentially too tired to push food through your band, so the food just sits there. But your esophagus is meant to be a conduit (or passage) from your mouth to your stomach; it is not meant to digest your food and is definitely not meant to hold food. Unlike tough stomach lining, the lining of the esophagus is easily irritated by food sitting around.

"IF FOOD IS JUST SITTING IN MY ESOPHAGUS, THEN WHY DON'T I FEEL PRESSURE OR RESTRICTION LIKE I USED TO?"

What happens if you bang your head against a wall? Initially you feel pain. What would happen if you kept banging your head against the wall? Eventually your forehead would go numb. This is what happens to your esophagus after you've had the band in place for a while. The band acts as a roadblock at the bottom of your esophagus, which initially senses it and sends pain signals to your brain, saying "Hey, there's a bad traffic jam down here. Stop eating!" You might sense this as a feeling of pressure, pain, or tightness. Many patients call it "restriction." Over time, however, your body realizes that it won't die from this roadblock, and rather than work hard to clear the obstruction, the tired esophagus lets the food sit there. The nerve fibers quit sending pain signals to your brain. Consequently, you no longer sense uncomfortable pressure and assume the stagnant food has passed through.

Sometimes a patient complains that she can eat a "whole hamburger, buns and all, Doc!" When using the barium swallow, I show her a pencil tip-sized channel opening through the band. I ask, "If the channel is only as wide as the tip of the pencil, how could a hamburger possibly go through?" The answer is that it cannot, even if she chews it really well. The hamburger is just sitting in her esophagus, causing damage. And sometimes, as I mentioned before, none of the barium goes through, indicating a total obstruction. If the patient is still not convinced, I give her the Cottage Cheese Test.

In this test, I take cottage cheese, a soft mushy food, and mix it with barium. The patient eats a small spoonful or two of the mixture. Using the fluoroscopy, I can show that this soft food is sitting above the band in the esophagus, meaning that tougher texture foods must also be sitting above the band. It is a powerful image of what is happening when she eats, so hopefully she will make better food choices rather than insisting on a tight, restrictive band.

Here is the image again of a dilated esophagus:

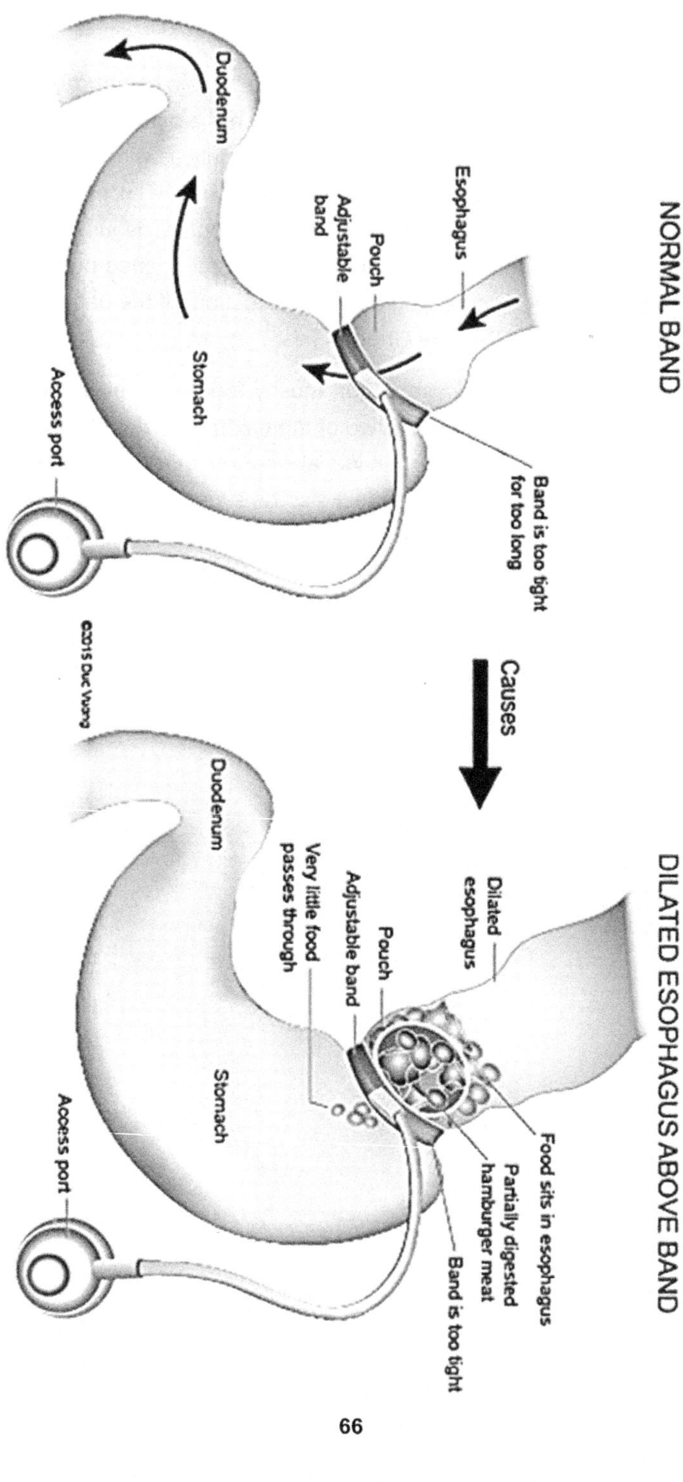
NORMAL BAND
Esophagus
Pouch
Adjustable band
Band is too tight for too long
Duodenum
Stomach
Access port
Causes
©2015 Duc Vuong
DILATED ESOPHAGUS ABOVE BAND
Dilated esophagus
Pouch
Adjustable band
Very little food passes through
Food sits in esophagus
Partially digested hamburger meat
Band is too tight
Duodenum
Stomach
Access port

Persistent Abdominal Pain at the Top of the Stomach/Bottom of the Chest—Persistent pain in this area (called the epigastrium), especially with fever or chills, is a serious sign of possible gastric band erosion. This means the band could have caused a hole in your stomach or esophagus. The best way to check this is to have an experienced bariatric surgeon perform an endoscopy. A gastroenterologist might not know some of the subtler signs of a band erosion, especially if the band is not visible. One time I saw an air bubble form around a skin fold right above a patient's band. I almost dismissed it until I saw a second air bubble come up from the same area, then a series of small air bubbles. This suggested some sort of unusual connection to the intraabdominal cavity, which meant the integrity of the stomach lining was compromised. In other words, there had to be a very small hole that was letting these air bubbles pass through! I almost missed this very subtle sign, and I do these endoscopies to look at bands all of the time. I removed this patient's band shortly thereafter.

Sometimes an eroded band shows up as an infected port, so you should know where your port is located. Some patients think their band is located where the port is placed, but this is not the case. Your port is underneath your skin and above your muscle, but your band is *internal*—around the top part of your stomach inside your abdominal cavity. Different surgeons will put the port in different locations; I have seen ports in the left upper quadrant, left lateral quadrant, right upper quadrant, around the belly button, and right below the xiphoid, which is the bone at the bottom of your sternum! If your port site feels warm to the touch, with red and "angry-looking" skin, and hurts when it is touched, you need to see a bariatric surgeon immediately for a barium swallow and/or an endoscopy. Even though these symptoms could indicate a port infection, a band erosion is also a possibility.

Summary and Tips: "Am I too TIGHT?"

1) Answer the questions and check the boxes that apply:

	YES	NO
Are you experiencing increasing heartburn or reflux?		
Do you have a nighttime cough that wakes you up?		
Is your asthma getting worse?		
Have you been diagnosed with pneumonia recently?		

Is food getting stuck more than once a month?

Two or more Yes's mean you need to make an appointment to see your bariatric surgeon for a possible DEFLATION.

2) How often are you burping up old food contents?

____

3) "My last appointment with a bariatric surgeon was...

____."

If the answer is more than 3 months ago, then you need to make another appointment.

7

Possible Band Complications

"Sometimes the problems that we create with surgery are worse than the diseases we are trying to treat." *– Dr. Kelvin Higa, Bariatric Surgery Pioneer*

If you are regaining weight or have stalled in your weight loss before reaching your goal, your surgeon's first objective is to make sure that there is nothing wrong with your band. This almost always requires diagnostic studies such as an EGD or barium swallow. "What could be wrong with my band?" you ask. Lots! And not just with your band, but also the gastric and esophageal tissues near it. The band is a mechanical device that requires close follow-up, regular check-ups, and maintenance, just like any other device. Here is a list of potential problems to watch out for. I will cover each in more detail.

1. Band leaks

2. Esophageal Dysfunction

3. Concentric Pouch Dilatation

4. Slips

5. Erosions

Band Leaks

If you regain weight, especially if you lose restriction quickly after a fill, you may have a leak in your band. The leak can occur anywhere along the device—from the port, to the tubing, to the actual balloon within the band itself. Leaks can also occur at anytime—at the time of surgery, years later, or anytime in between. The US Clinical Trial that granted Allergan FDA approval for the Lap-Band quoted a 2% port leak rate at 3 years.

"DIAGNOSING A LEAK COULD INVOLVE SEVERAL OFFICE VISITS."

Diagnosing a leak could involve several office visits, so don't get frustrated. In order to make this diagnosis, your surgeon or bariatric team must first *suspect* a leak, and they will only suspect a leak if you keep returning complaining of lack of restriction. However, since a loss of restriction may stem from a dilated esophagus, to make a proper diagnosis, they must keep accurate records of your fill volume. I tell my patients it is important that they know approximately how much fluid should be in their band. **Always ask your provider how much fluid is in your band, then WRITE IT DOWN.** Some programs will aspirate out the fluid in your band every time to check the volume, but not always, and therefore a patient's awareness of her fill volume could help the bariatric team diagnose a leak more quickly. An upper GI or barium swallow (sometimes repeated a few times) will show whether the band is less tight than previously documented.

"THE COMBINATION OF LACK OF RESTRICTION AND DECREASING SALINE AMOUNTS IS IMPORTANT TO DIAGNOSING BAND LEAKS."

Once a leak is suspected from routine tracking of band fill volumes, the surgeon has to CONFIRM it, usually by aspirating all of the fluid out of the band and then measuring a precise amount of fluid. At this time, I also like to add a biocompatible (nontoxic) blue dye to the fluid. The blue dye confirms that I'm definitely accessing the port next time I go to measure the amount of fluid in the band. It will also aid in the location of a leak at the time of surgery. Another option is to add a radiopaque contrast material to the fluid and use a fluoroscope, which is a type of x-ray machine, to see if it leaks out, but this requires equipment that is not always available and may not reveal a leak too slow to show up on the X-Ray.

If these methods do not immediately show a leak, I have the patient return in one month to have the fluid remeasured. "Why do I have to wait one month?" Leaks can be VERY SLOW, so it could take one month or more for there to be a noticeable difference in the fluid volume. If I remove as little as 1 cc less than the amount that should have been in the band, there is a leak. Slow leaks take two or more months to confirm, as well as several office visits (and associated costs) to diagnose, so you must be *persistent and consistent* with the follow-up plan and as informed as possible about your band fluid levels.

Fixing a leak requires another surgery. If you have had your band for a few years, the leak is most likely in the tubing itself. If the leak is near the port, then often just the port and a short segment of tubing need to be replaced. But sometimes, the entire band might need to be replaced, especially if the leak is in the balloon portion of the band. Sometimes, however, it is not possible to know where the leak is prior to surgery.

If you are faced with a leak in your band—especially if you are struggling with your weight loss or if you don't like the need for adjustments—you might consider revising the band to a different surgery. I go into revisions later in the book.

Esophageal Dysfunction

As I discussed in previous sections, esophageal dysfunction means that the esophagus is no longer working properly and is potentially very serious. You do not want a nonfunctioning esophagus; just ask people who suffer from esophageal cancer or esophageal dysmotility disorders like achalasia or nutcracker esophagus. They will tell you how miserable having a nonfunctioning or poorly functioning esophagus can be. A barium swallow is the best ways to diagnose this, and again, such tests should be done with the surgeon watching. If your surgeon cannot be present, ask for a CD of the images that you can take to your surgeon.

I find it helpful when an adopted patient (someone who had surgery by a different surgeon) comes to see me with a disk of her images in hand, not just a radiologist's report. I watch for flow down a smooth esophagus and easy passage through a properly angled band. I look out for a dilated, twisted, or spastic esophagus. Sometimes the esophagus is curved like a backwards letter "c," indicating an advanced condition needing immediate attention.

Surgeons believe that deflating the band will allow most of the dysfunction to resolve, but this is not always the outcome. Sometimes the band has to be removed completely and the esophagus reassessed a few months later. If the esophagus is still not working properly, you might no longer be a candidate for ANY weight loss surgery. The best way to avoid this scenario is through regular follow-up with your surgeon. If you start having problems like frequent sticking or heartburn, you should call your surgeon immediately for an appointment.

Concentric Pouch Dilatation

In dilatation, the small stomach pouch above the band starts to dilate or stretch out, which is visible on a barium swallow. Surgeons agree that a concentric pouch dilatation is the first step to a band slippage. As the pouch expands, it pulls the stomach tissue up over the band, eventually leading to a slip. My clinic is aggressive about treating pouch dilatations, and I deflate the band at the first indication. After deflation, the patient consumes nothing but liquids for two weeks. Most of the time, this resolves pouch dilatation, but not always. Don't assume that everything is better because the surgeon deflated the band or because you can eat again. Come back for your post-deflation follow-up, because the next problem could still happen.

Band Slippage

In a slipped band, a portion of the stomach tissue pulls up and over the band, where it bunches and flops. It looks much like the beret cap of an army officer or a stereotypical Frenchman. The extra stomach tissue could flop over the band towards the front of your belly wall (an anterior slip, the most common direction) or towards your spine (a posterior slip). A barium swallow will show that the slipped band is angled wrong on the X-ray. Instead of being at the proper 45-degree angle tilt, the band will be horizontal (an anterior slip) or will look like a circle (a posterior slip.) I have also seen slips where the band was angled properly, but the barium pooled above the band. It is important that your surgeon be present during the X-ray study because a radiologist might not be familiar enough with bands to recognize the various indications of a slippage.

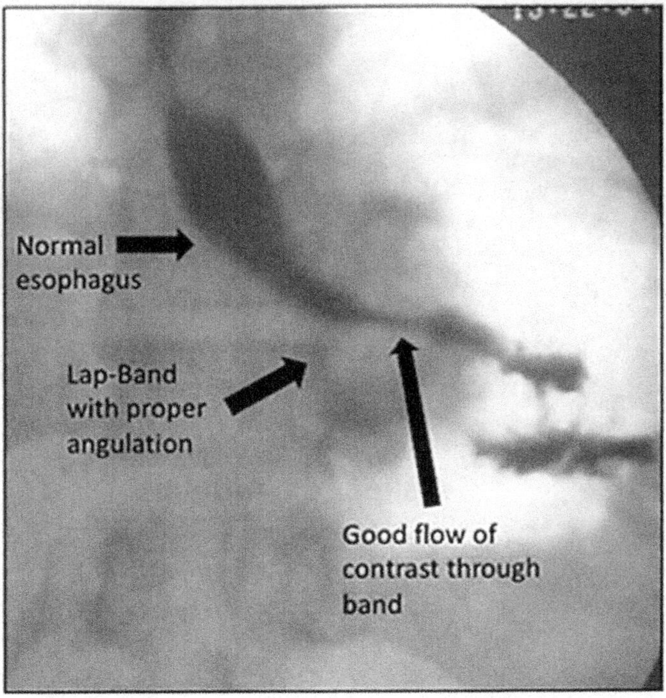

Normal Band Appearance: The band is a rectangular shadow, angled approximately 45 degrees.

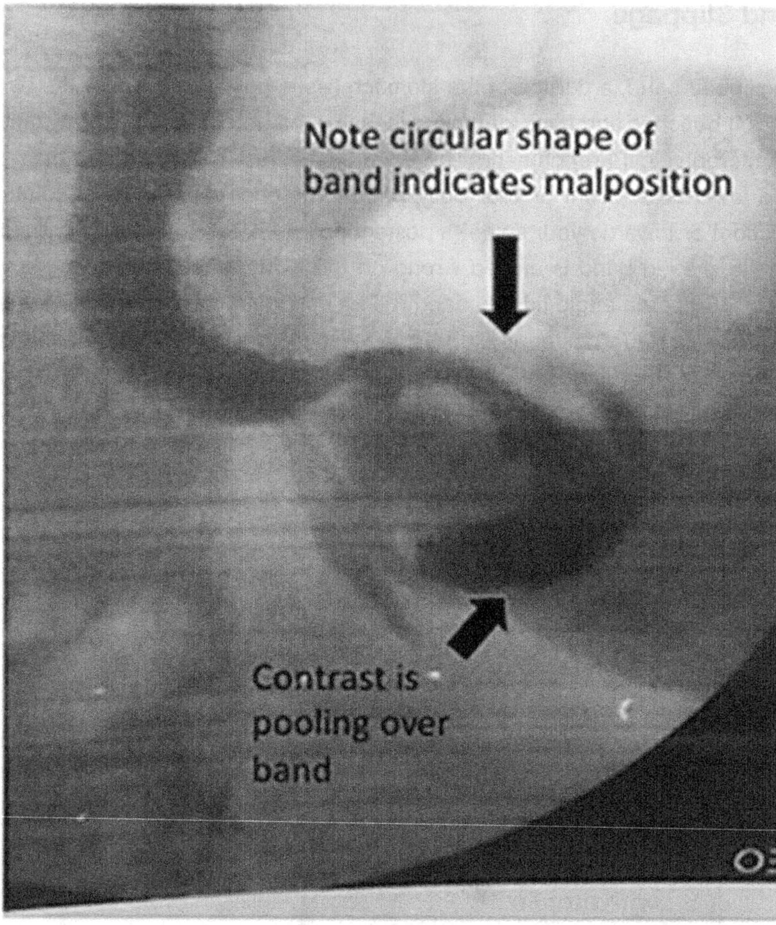

A slipped band

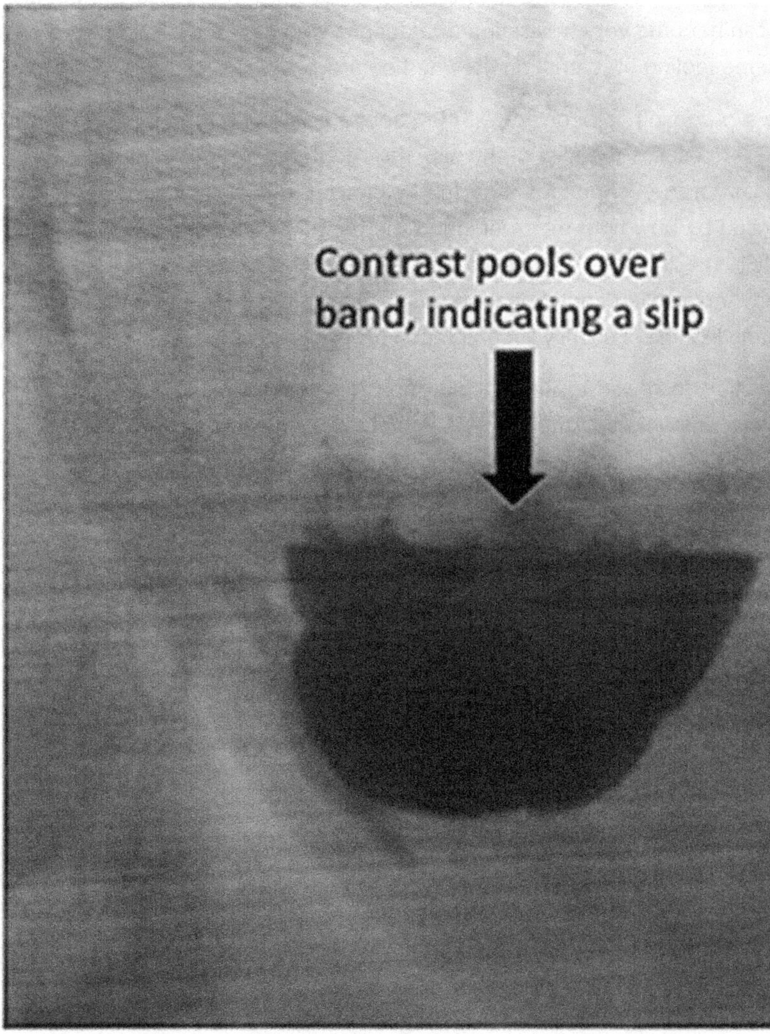

Contrast sitting in a blind pouch above the band indicates a slip.

Assuming the absence of serious signs of sepsis, the treatment for a slip is to deflate the band completely and immediately, to consume only liquids for 2-4 weeks, and to remain patient. Usually the extra stomach tissue falls back down into its proper place with this relatively simple treatment, in which case you can be readjusted *slowly*; however, once a band slips, it has a tendency to reslip, especially as the fill volume gets close to what it was when the slip occurred. This can become very frustrating for patients, who may not be able to return to the same feeling of restriction they had before.

If the slip doesn't self-correct with the above treatment, then I usually perform an EGD to assess the size of the slip, the "tightness" of the band opening, the condition of the esophagus, and the health of the gastric tissues. Often I am surprised by how tight the opening of the band is when completely deflated—this tells me that the chance of reinflation will be low, since the tissues are already too swollen and "bunched up" to allow the band to work properly. In a scenario like this, I usually recommend surgery to remove and revise the band.

The option to revise to another surgery depends on many factors, including your current weight (American insurance companies require that you have a BMI >35 with a comorbidity or BMI>40), your financial situation, your preferences, and your surgeon and clinic. **However, the final decision of whether or not to have another surgery ultimately rests with you!** Most surgeons today prefer to revise to a different surgery than to reposition the band. I prefer to revise to a sleeve if the patient was successful with the band, because patients have good results and I can usually perform the band removal and revision in one surgery. I discuss this more later in the book.

Often a slipped band that is not causing ANY problems can remain deflated for a long time, thereby avoiding an unnecessary procedure for the patient. However, this tactic does carry some risk, as the unproblematic slip can become an "acute" slip. In an acute slip, the stomach tissues that pass through the band have become so swollen or bunched up that nothing passes through, which can compromise blood flow through the stomach and cause stomach tissues to start dying. This causes significant abdominal pain and vomiting. This slip has now become the surgical emergency of my patient John that I described earlier, and the bariatric surgeon will likely take the patient to surgery immediately to assess the situation. Depending on what he finds, he might remove the band completely, unbuckle the band, or reposition the band. I would remove the band completely, but some surgeons will decide differently. I encourage you to express to your surgeon whether your preference is to remove the band or to try to salvage the band.

Erosion—Cases in which part of the band has eroded into your stomach (the band has "eaten" its way *into* your stomach) are rare but serious. Most patients with an eroded band have severe abdominal pain and may develop an infection causing severe illness.

Erosion often presents as an infection around the port site, which is seen on a CT scan as inflammation of the tissues around the port. A barium swallow could show that contrast passes around a band or over a band instead of through the band. Sometimes radiologists miss this subtle appearance, so you need an experienced surgeon to watch the X-ray.

Maria's Story

My patient, Maria, had successfully lost weight with her band, but had it deflated because she was pregnant. Once her son was 18 months old, she came back to my office weighing the same as when she was originally deflated. She came in to have her band filled, because she was ready to start losing weight again, and she had no symptoms of complications. I performed a routine barium swallow and discovered that her band was sitting at the wrong angle, although the barium went through. I asked her to rotate and drink contrast multiple times, and from a side view, I could see the contrast flow *over* her band and into her stomach, meaning that her band was partially inside her stomach! I'm not sure a well-trained radiologist would have found this erosion, because the radiographic sign was very slight. I'm not sure why I kept looking. Was it because I have performed hundreds of such tests and trusted my "doctor's instinct" even though everything seemed fine at first glance? Maybe I just got lucky. I'm not sure. Either way, Maria had her band removed a few weeks later.

If the erosion is slow, as in the above case, your body could potentially seal off the infection so that you don't become very sick or sick for long. One patient of mine was completely asymptomatic except for some weight regain, and her barium swallow showed normal passage through the band. Yet an EGD showed that the band was mostly eroded through the stomach wall. Upon closer review of her medical history, the patient had had repeated episodes of abdominal pain in the past year that gradually got better over time or once the band was deflated. I have also spoken to surgeons who have had patients with completely eroded gastric bands that pass out of the body through either stool or vomit. I am astonished that a gastric band can make it through 18-20 feet of bowel! Sometimes the band will get stuck at the end of the small bowel and cause a blockage. This requires a surgery to remove, and in some cases even an open laparotomy to repair.

Surgeons used to think that band erosions were rare (occurring in less than 1% of band patients), but now with more years of data, the rate of erosion could be as high as 5%, which is 1 in 20 cases! This means there are potentially many gastric band patients who are at risk. In 2013 a study out of Australia with 15 years of follow-up showed a 3.4% erosion rate (O'Brien, 2013.)

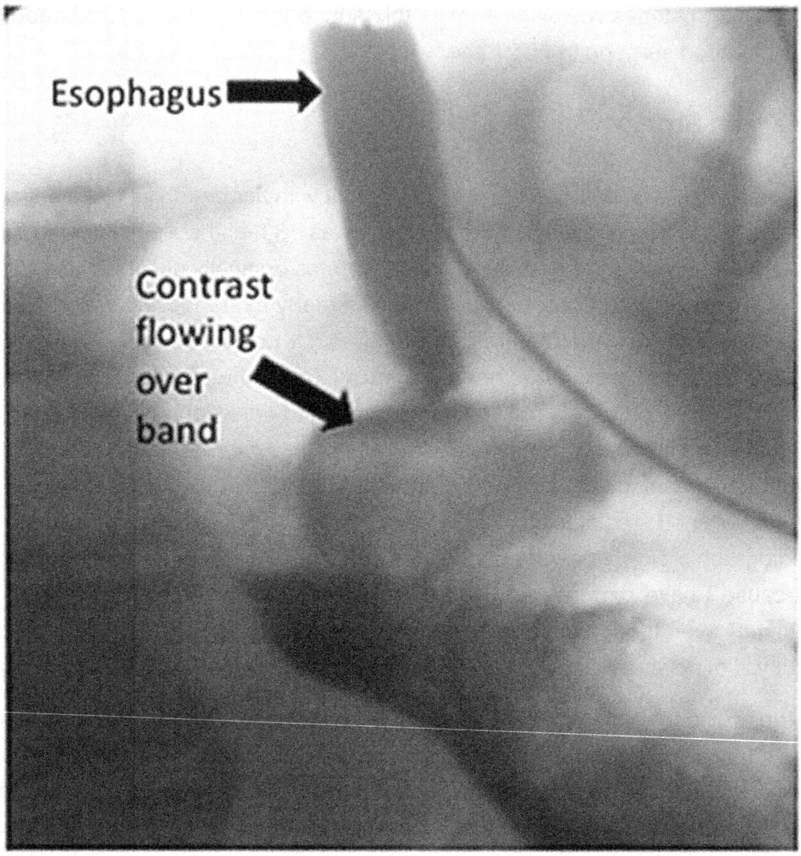

Band Erosion: Contrast is flowing over the band, indicating that a portion of the band is inside of the stomach.

As frightening as these scenarios seem, most of them are reversible and fixable. Find a good bariatric surgeon that you trust and connect into a patient-oriented bariatric program.

Summary and Tips: "Have I ever SEEN my Band?"

1) Run your fingers along the bottom of your rib cage on both sides until they meet in the middle. The bone there is the xiphoid process, which is at the bottom of your sternum. Move your finger up one inch. That is where your Lap-Band is! You can confirm this placement by requesting a barium swallow and waving your finger over your xiphoid, and it will correlate with the live image on the X-Ray screen.

2) Have you ever had a barium swallow during an adjustment?

YES NO

3) Have you had an endoscopy (EGD) since having your band placed?

YES NO

4) How much fluid is in your band? ______________________________

8

Technical Considerations of Revisional Surgery

"It is our attitude at the beginning of a difficult task which, more than anything else, will affect its successful outcome." *– William James*

The technical aspects of performing revisional surgery might seem unimportant, tedious, or not of concern, but if you spend some time with this section, you not only will appreciate your surgeon's skill in performing your revision safely, you will also relieve many of his concerns when he realizes that he is speaking to a knowledgeable patient. This should peak your interest enough to read ahead!

"REVISIONAL SURGERY OFTEN EQUALS TWO SURGERIES."

Prepare yourself for the fact that your revision surgery might require two separate procedures—one to remove your band and another to revise it to the procedure you and your surgeon decide is best. Most European surgeons will do two separate procedures, because some studies indicate a possible decrease in the risk of complications, described below.

Complications Possibly Avoided by Two-Stage Surgery

Adhesions:

The Band can cause significant adhesions (scar tissue) around the top portion of the stomach, where the new pouch (be it a sleeve or bypass pouch) needs to go. The surgeon needs to dissect out this scar tissue in order to see and access the stomach's anatomy, and hence safely perform the revisional surgery. Most of the time, this scar tissue is soft and filmy, but sometimes it is quite dense, making the dissection treacherous.

The band itself can be densely adhered to the liver, sometimes even "buried" in the liver. The process of dissecting the band out in such cases could cause a lot of blood loss from the liver, which makes the surgery longer and harder.

The band can also be adhered to other nearby organs, like the spleen or diaphragm. Dissecting the band from spleen may cause bleeding, and because bleeding from the spleen can be rapid, the spleen might need to be taken out. This is called a splenectomy.

In the initial surgery to insert the band, some surgeons suture a portion of the stomach over the band and onto the crus of the diaphragm to try to prevent band slips. Such suturing might or might not accomplish this goal, but it definitely makes removal of the band much harder because the band adheres to the crus of the diaphragm, very close to the esophagus. No surgeon wants to cause a hole in the esophagus because its high location and two-layer musculature makes it difficult to repair.

Taking down these adhesions could take an hour or more, which in some cases is the typical time it takes to do a primary weight loss surgery.

Dislodgement of the Band:

Don't assume the band is always where it is supposed to be. Sometimes the band is dislodged in unusual places, like next to the heart in the chest cavity, inside the stomach, or in the intestines. Such dislodgements can make the surgery very difficult and dangerous, so your surgery might convert from laparoscopic (the less invasive method that uses a tiny camera and instruments inserted through one or two small incisions) to open (the method of cutting open the abdomen). If the band is not where it should be, the surgeon most likely will not revise you in one surgery because it would be stressful on your body and require a lengthy recovery period.

Possibility of an open procedure:

Depending on what the surgeon finds and his level of experience, you might end up needing an open surgery. Sometimes open surgery can help figure out what has happened to the band and your anatomy. Sometimes it is necessary if you are in critical condition or septic. The difference in recovery times between open and laparoscopic surgery can be significant.

Esophageal considerations:

I have encountered a few unpleasant occasions in which I discovered that the band was placed on or very near to the esophagus. The esophagus is a different organ from the stomach with a different anatomical make-up. Unlike the stomach, which has three muscle layers, the esophagus has only two layers—this makes it more difficult to repair if the surgeon causes a hole in it. Also, the aorta (the largest blood vessel that delivers blood from your heart to the rest of your body) runs right under the esophagus. There are actually many critical structures in the esophageal area, including the left and right vagus nerves, the thoracic duct, and the recurrent laryngeal nerve, to name a few. When the band is near the esophagus, then, the surgeon needs to proceed very carefully to avoid damaging these multiple structures.

Uncertainty of how the band was placed:

While the major steps of gastric band placement are uniform, there are a few minor variations. During the early period of Lap-Band surgery, surgeons used the "pars gastric" technique that placed the band a little lower on the stomach. This technique had a high slip rate, so surgeons switched to the "pars flaccida" technique, which meant the band was placed higher and with minimal dissection. This technique has better outcomes, and this is how most surgeons were trained to place the band. Most surgeons will perform what is called a "gastro-gastric plication" and stitch the floppy part of the stomach to the new smaller stomach pouch above the band in order to keep the band from slipping. As I mentioned earlier, some surgeons might stitch the stomach to the crus of the diaphragm for the same reason. The number of sutures placed and the instruments used to tie down the sutures also vary. Some surgeons use a knot-forming device in which a metal clip secures the sutures. During a revisional surgery, such clips can get in the way of the stapler. I heard of one surgeon who "oversewed" the bottom half of the stomach with a nondissolvable suture in an attempt to make the stomach smaller and supposedly improve weight loss. The variation in techniques and materials used in placing the band therefore influence how your surgeon performs the revision and how complex the revision will be.

Placement of a feeding tube:

Depending on the severity of the damage caused by band complications or the removal surgery, you might need a feeding tube, especially if the surgeon anticipates that you will need to be kept NPO (nothing by mouth) for a period of time. He will place this small tube into either your stomach or small intestine and out through your skin. It serves as a conduit by which you are given some nutrition, such as protein shakes, because nutrition is necessary to heal from the surgery. This is far more common during emergency surgeries than during elective band revisions.

Placement of drains:

Most of the time small drains are placed as a precaution, but some cases require multiple large drains. Drains help control infection (in cases of intraabdominal catastrophes that require an open procedure) or detect early complications like leaks. When I first started doing band revisions, I always placed a small drain that I would remove in my office the following week. Often, the patient would complain about pain from the drain more than from the actual surgery itself. So I now place a drain only if I'm concerned about something or if the revision surgery was more difficult than expected. However, some surgeons always place drains during a revision surgery, and that is completely in keeping with surgical standards.

Increased risk of complications:

Many small studies indicate that revisional surgeries are fraught with much higher rates of complications than are primary surgeries. Some complications are minor (increased wound infections and readmissions for dehydration, for example), but there also appears to be a much higher rate of serious complications, such as staple line leaks. In the case of revision to sleeve, the leak rate can be as high as 4%, while primary sleeve leak rates are around 1%. The same appears true for revisional surgery to gastric bypass. Fortunately as of the time of writing of this book, I have not had one revisional leak. I hope that rate continues!

****

The eight factors above create a large variability in operating time, which can disrupt the flow of the OR schedule, affect the remaining surgical patients waiting for their surgeries, and wreak havoc on the surgeon's mental clarity. But simply removing the Band (which is not always simple) can usually be accomplished in around 30-60 minutes. Three to six months later, at the time of the revisional surgery, there is usually less scar tissue, and the surgery is similar to a primary surgery in terms of difficulty and operative duration. Some studies from Germany suggest a decreased rate of leaks with this approach. Knowing these factors, revising the band in two stages has significant appeal.

Single-Stage vs. Two-Stage Revision

In contrast to the European surgeons, some American surgeons (including myself) always *try* to perform revisions in only one surgery. It is difficult for a patient to undergo two separate surgeries: two anesthesia inductions, two dissections, two recoveries, and two separate medical bills. There is no clear answer as to whether two-stage or single-stage revisional surgery is better. **I think it depends on the patient's particular circumstances and the surgeon's skill with revisions; together these two factors will determine which revision procedure will be performed and how.** Ask your surgeon how many revisional surgeries he has done and what his preferences are.

Unfortunately, revisional surgeries will become more and more common in the near future, not because of higher band failure rates, but because weight loss surgery is becoming more common. Inadequate weight loss or weight regain after surgery is regularly as high as 30% and possibly as high as 50% if the initial BMI is >50. The professional surgical societies and medical industry have started offering more courses for surgeons on how to approach revisions. **My stance has always been that we need to place more emphasis on proper preoperative education to avoid these revisions in the first place.**

9

Nonsurgical Options

"You gain strength, courage, and confidence by every experience in which you really stop to look fear in the face. You are able to say to yourself, 'I lived through this horror. I can take the next thing that comes along.'" – *Eleanor Roosevelt, former First Lady of the United States* aMaybe you're not ready to go under the knife again, your insurance won't cover revisional surgery, or you've lost your insurance all together. Maybe you haven't quite exhausted all avenues toward weight loss with your band. Or maybe my description of the technical aspects of revisional surgery has caused you to have second thoughts. In this section, I will discuss available nonsurgical options, namely pharmaceuticals and meal-replacement programs.

Pharmaceuticals, aka Diet Pills

You might be thinking, "Not so fast, Dr. V. I did not go through weight loss surgery just to get back on diet pills again!" I understand that the thought of diet pills might seem counterintuitive for many WLS patients, but pharmaceuticals are an option for many patients who are struggling with their surgery, and not just gastric band surgery. Some practices use them to help struggling bypass and sleeve patients, too. Diet pills might be the jumpstart you need to get going again or the net you need to cushion your freefall, and they seem to work differently once a patient has had surgery. Patients who meet the following criteria fall within the current recommended guidelines for the use of diet pills, which should ALWAYS be used in combination with a diet and exercise regimen:

- BMI=30 kg/m2 or greater (obese) or
- BMI=27 kg/m2 or greater (overweight) in the presence of at least one weight-related comorbidity such as hypertension, type-II diabetes mellitus, or dyslipidemia

Many diseases require more than one option to treat, such as diabetes. If one diabetes medication does not work, physicians know to add a second medication. If the second medication does not work, they consider adding insulin to your regimen. That is THREE modalities to treat one disease. Yet for some reason, if a patient gets incomplete results from ONE weight loss surgery, she and the surgery are labeled failures.

"WE NEED TO GET AWAY FROM THE IDEA THAT WEIGHT LOSS SURGERY IS EITHER A "SUCCESS" OR A "FAILURE."

I believe that we bariatric surgeons should use all of the weapons in our armamentarium including pharmaceuticals to fight this illness, I also believe that we should use them sooner rather than later, at the earliest signs that the patient is struggling, rather than waiting until the patient has regained weight. Here are some of the options I provide in my clinic:

Phentermine:

First approved by the Food and Drug Administration (FDA) in 1959, Phentermine (Adipex-P, Suprenza, Ionamin®) is an amphetamine-like prescription medication used to suppress appetite by triggering the release of the brain chemical norepinephrine. Norepinephrine increases the blood's concentrations of the appetite-regulating hormone leptin, which decreases your hunger or makes you feel full longer. It is approved only for short-term use—12 weeks or less—because it may become addictive. Phentermine is the most commonly prescribed prescription appetite suppressant, partly because it's significantly cheaper than the other major FDA-approved diet drugs. But phentermine has some unpleasant side effects, such as increased blood pressure, dizziness, dry mouth, sleeplessness, nervousness, and constipation.

Phentermine is probably most notable for being the "Phen" in the Fen-Phen or Dexfen-Phen of the mid 1990's, which drew much scrutiny after reports that these drugs, when used in combination, caused increased risk of heart valve damage. The "Fen" (Fenfluramine) and the "Dexfen" (Dexfenfluramine) never received FDA approval in combination with Phentermine, and the FDA removed them from the market. The reports did not indicate that Phentermine caused any heart damage when used alone.

Qsymia (phentermine/topiramate):

FDA-approved in 2012, Qsymia combines phentermine (described above) with topiramate extended release, both of which had previously been approved for use on their own. Topiramate is a seizure and migraine drug that causes weight loss in several ways, including increasing feelings of fullness, making foods taste less appealing, and increasing calorie burning. Studies on Qsymia show a 1-year weight loss of 9-14% of body weight, depending on the dose.

Belviq (locaserin):

Around the same time it approved Qsymia in 2012, the FDA also approved Belviq (lorcaserin hydrochloride). Belviq might be an option for patients who cannot tolerate the side effects of phentermine. Studies show that treatment with Belviq for up to one year is associated with an average weight loss ranging from 3 percent to 3.7 percent. Belviq works by activating the serotonin 2C receptor in the brain, which may help a person eat less and feel full after eating smaller amounts of food.

At dosages intended for weight loss, Belviq does not significantly turn on the different serotonin switches responsible for the effects of hallucinogens (such as LSD) and addictive drugs. The seratonin 2C receptor, however, is the same one implicated in the Fen-Phen controversy. According to Belviq's official website:

> In 1997, the weight-loss drugs fenfluramine and dexfenfluramine were withdrawn from the market after evidence emerged that they caused heart valve damage. This effect is assumed to be related to activation of the serotonin 2B receptor on heart tissue. When used at the approved dose of 10 milligrams twice a day, Belviq does not appear to activate the serotonin 2B receptor.
>
> Heart valve function was assessed by echocardiography in nearly 8,000 patients in the Belviq development program. There was no statistically significant difference in the development of FDA-defined valve abnormalities between Belviq and placebo-treated patients. Because preliminary data suggest that the number of serotonin 2B receptors may be increased in patients with congestive heart failure, Belviq should be used with caution in patients with this condition. Belviq has not been studied in patients with serious valvular heart disease (www.belviqhcp.com).

The safety and efficacy of Belviq were evaluated in three randomized, placebo-controlled trials that included nearly 8,000 obese and overweight patients, with and without type 2 diabetes, who were treated for 52 to 104 weeks. All participants also received a reduced calorie diet and exercise counseling. This is a thorough test, but because the longterm effects of Belviq are not yet known, please discuss this option carefully with your healthcare provider.

Contrave (Buproprion/Naltrexone):

In 2014, the FDA approved Contrave, which is a combination of naltrexone and bupropion in an extended-release form. On their own, naltrexone treats alcohol and opioid dependence, and bupropion treats depression, seasonal affective disorder, and smoking dependence. Results from a clinical trial showed that over one year, patients had an average weight loss of 4.1%, with 42% of patients losing at least 5% percent of their body weight.

Saxenda (liraglutide):

In December 2014, shortly after its approval of Contrave, the FDA approved Saxenda (liraglutide). Saxenda contains the same active ingredient as Victoza, a drug used to treat type-II diabetes, but at different doses (3 mg and 1.8 mg, respectively). However, Saxenda is not indicated for the treatment of type-II diabetes. Clinical trials with patients without diabetes showed an average weight loss of 4.5%, and 62% lost at least 5%of their body weight.

****

After a 13-year period of no weight loss drug approvals, the FDA approved four new weight loss drugs in a short two-year span. This underscores the recognition of the ever-increasing battle against obesity and the medical industry's attempt to fight it. Could it also indicate the U.S. government's view of the importance of obesity treatment?

These pharmaceuticals may be a way to kick-start your weight loss. I also use them to help my band patients while they are deflated or any weight loss surgery patient who is struggling. However, as with most diet pills, once you stop taking them, you might regain the weight you lost. That's why they need to be part of a plan that includes healthy eating and regular exercise—you're more likely to maintain your weight loss over time if you don't rely solely on medications (or surgery, for that matter).

Meal-Replacement Programs

Complete meal replacement programs must be monitored by a physician, unlike commercially-available supplement products, such as Slimfast or Herbalife. The typical complete meal replacement program will last upwards of 6 months, with a three-month period of exclusive product usage (no consumption of "real" food) followed by a transitional phase during which food is slowly reintroduced into your diet as supplement consumption tapers down. A meal replacement program conducted in this manner can eliminate 20-30% of total body weight. Of course there are other, less strict variations, but these might not yield the same results. The medical field is not sure how this will work long-term after weight loss surgery, but I have used this strategy with some of my struggling patients with good results, at least in the short term. The monitoring includes regular blood work and weekly educational groups, which ensure the safety and health of the patient and contribute to long-term success.

My surgical philosophy is that pharmaceuticals and meal-replacements are safe and effective only as part of a comprehensive bariatrics program and should be considered "rescue" options for patients struggling with weight regain. We need many "bullets in our holster" to fight the complex disease of obesity. While some primary care providers see only weight loss surgery "failures" and conclude that weight loss surgery does not work, multiple studies show that weight loss surgery is the best option for long-term weight loss success and the elimination of associated comorbidities. Weight loss surgery is not perfect (that might be why you're reading this book), but it's the best we have and is more effective when used in combination with other treatments, such as diet, exercise, and pharmaceuticals. Not all surgeons agree with this or have interest in pharmaceuticals or meal replacement programs, so check with your surgeon to see if he or his clinic offers these services. Often surgeons partner with a local bariatrician who offers these treatment plans.

Summary and Tips: "Have I REALLY tried EVERYTHING?"

1) Pharmaceuticals might be the jump start you need to get back on track. Call your bariatric surgeon or doctor to see if you are a candidate for a diet pill to curb your appetite while you reassess your food choices.

2) Start keeping a food journal now because diet pills will be more effective if you change what you are eating.

3) Have you tried a physician-supervised meal replacement program? Google "Optifast" and see if there are programs in your area.

10

Surgical Revision Options

"When written in Chinese, the word 'crisis' is composed of two characters. One represents danger and the other represents opportunity." *– John F. Kennedy, former U.S. President*

"I am throwing in the towel with the Band. What are my options?" Maybe you've had enough. You've reached your wit's end. Your friend just had a sleeve or bypass, and she is doing much better, losing weight faster, and not struggling with repeated adjustments or complications. Maybe you are wondering, "Is there something better?"

The decision whether or not to keep your gastric band is personal. **If you decide to proceed with a revisional surgery, do not feel that you are a failure.** Obesity is a complicated disease. That is why there are many surgical weight loss options.

"DO NOT VIEW YOUR SURGERY AS A FAILURE, BUT RATHER AS INADEQUATE OR INCOMPLETE TREATMENT."

As I suggested earlier, think of obesity like hypertension or diabetes. Many patients require insulin in addition to oral diabetes medicines or more than one antihypertensive medicine, and we don't consider them "failures." Think of a surgery that did not help you achieve a healthy weight as incomplete treatment. For example, some of my patients have lost 100 pounds with the band, but now their weight loss has stalled and they remain obese. The band has done its part, which was to help the patient get to a healthier weight and reduce the perioperative risk of a second surgery. The band was not a failure, but rather only a part of the treatment. This section will discuss some of the revision options available for gastric band patients. But first, three very important points:

1. This revision might not be the only surgery you need—As I discussed previously, your revisional surgery might be done in two stages, one to remove the band and one to perform the revision itself. But the second weight loss surgery might *still* be an incomplete treatment. If you look hard enough, you will always be able to find a surgeon to operate on you, but that does not mean another surgery is right for you. I have heard anecdotes of patients getting their fourth or fifth weight loss surgeries. I am not sure what their situations were, but having so many revisional surgeries seems like a high price to pay for something that clearly needs a different kind of supplemental treatment, such as nutritional modifications, psychological counseling, or perhaps even a surgery on a knee to make walking feasible. Some institutions seem to agree. In England, the medical system will pay for one weight loss surgery, making revisional surgery difficult to cover. Luckily in America, we do not have this limitation, but it might not be long before it happens.

2. Effective weight loss is not guaranteed—Good evidence of the long-term efficacy of revisional bariatric surgery currently does not exist. Early data seem to suggest that revisional surgery patients will catch up to their counterparts who had only the second surgery. In other words, in the short term, the medical profession has found that a patient with a band to sleeve revision will lose as much weight on average as a patient who had a sleeve to begin with. This is good news. However, we are not sure if the *long-term* weight loss results will be the same. Bariatric surgeons currently do not agree (or know) which revisional surgery is most effective after gastric banding. The medical literature currently is too sparse. I am an avid proponent for the sleeve gastrectomy, meaning I prefer revisions from band to sleeve, but I do not have any long-term scientific evidence to prove that this is the most effective revision. I just know that my band to sleeve revision patients love their sleeves more than they ever did the band, and their weight loss results are very good so far. Your surgeon(s) might prefer a gastric bypass or something else. But I believe that *preoperative education* is the key to weight loss surgery success!

3. You must be a very active participant in your revisional surgery—Revisional surgery is not like your first surgery. It demands that you come prepared and armed with information (one of the many reasons I wrote this book). You have to help your surgeon decide your best chance for success, and honesty about your struggles with the band is essential. If you have a sweet tooth, tell him that sweets have been a big part of your struggle, which might suggest that a revision to a gastric bypass would work best. If you enjoy fruits and vegetables but haven't been able to eat them because of the band, let your team know, because a sleeve would probably be right for you. Most importantly, you have to be honest with yourself. This is the time to look in the mirror and ask, "Do I really want to go through this again? What can I do to make sure that this is really the last time?"

Surgical Options

Deflate the Band and Leave It in Place

Even though this is technically not a surgery, I include it here because it is an option that can be effective. I've done this for several patients who have had a slip or dilated esophagus, especially if they are close to a normal BMI. I deflate the band completely, place them on liquids, and then my clinic and I teach them how to make proper food choices. Our clinic promotes a primarily pescatarian diet, which is a diet high in fresh fruits and vegetables, salads, whole grains, beans, tofu, fish, and seafood. We avoid red meats, dairy, breads, and processed foods. Eating this way enables patients to lose weight if they are still obese or maintain their weight if they have achieved a healthy weight. I also see these patients *regularly* to make sure nothing has changed with the band and check whether the slip or the dilated esophagus has resolved.

Only Remove the Band

As frightening as this might sound, some patients opt to have the band removed and NOT undergo another weight loss surgery. **You should *never* feel like you *must* have a "tool" to keep you from gaining weight.** You might decide that it is too risky or that it is not worth the cost and recovery time. You might decide to try it "the old-fashioned way." You might just be sick and tired of it all. This is a personal journey, and you should never feel pressured by anyone, not even your surgeon, to have another weight loss surgery. But you should be aware that the vast majority of gastric band patients who have the band removed without undergoing another surgery will regain weight in the long term (Aarts, E.O., et. Al, 2014.)

Re-band

Depending on your situation, a re-band might be an option, especially if you have been successful with your band but have a slip, tubing leak, or if you have an older type of band (Riele WW, et al, 2014.) In 2008, the manufacturer Allergan introduced the AP Lap-Band, changing the original band design to one that is wider with more balloon coverage area. Theoretically this should help with the feeling of restriction. The AP band also has different fill volumes than the old bands, giving surgeons a wider range for adjustments. The AP band has never been released in Mexico, so if you had your band placed in Mexico even after 2008, you have the old type of band. The new band is also easier for surgeons to unbuckle, which helps them reposition it. In the case of a slipped band, some dedicated band surgeons unbuckle the band but leave it in place and rebuckle it 3 months later when the scar tissue has reorganized. This seems like a lot of surgery to me—I can only imagine what it is like for the patient!

Most surgeons agree, however, that there are better revision options than fixing an existing band or replacing it with a newer model. Weight loss surgery is about balancing Risk and Reward. While the gastric band has an impressive safety profile, it is also one of the least powerful surgical weight loss options. I do not typically revise a band to another band because I believe that struggling band patients need a more powerful surgery. You must discuss this with your surgeon, do your homework, and decide what is right for you.

Revise the Band to the Gastric Sleeve

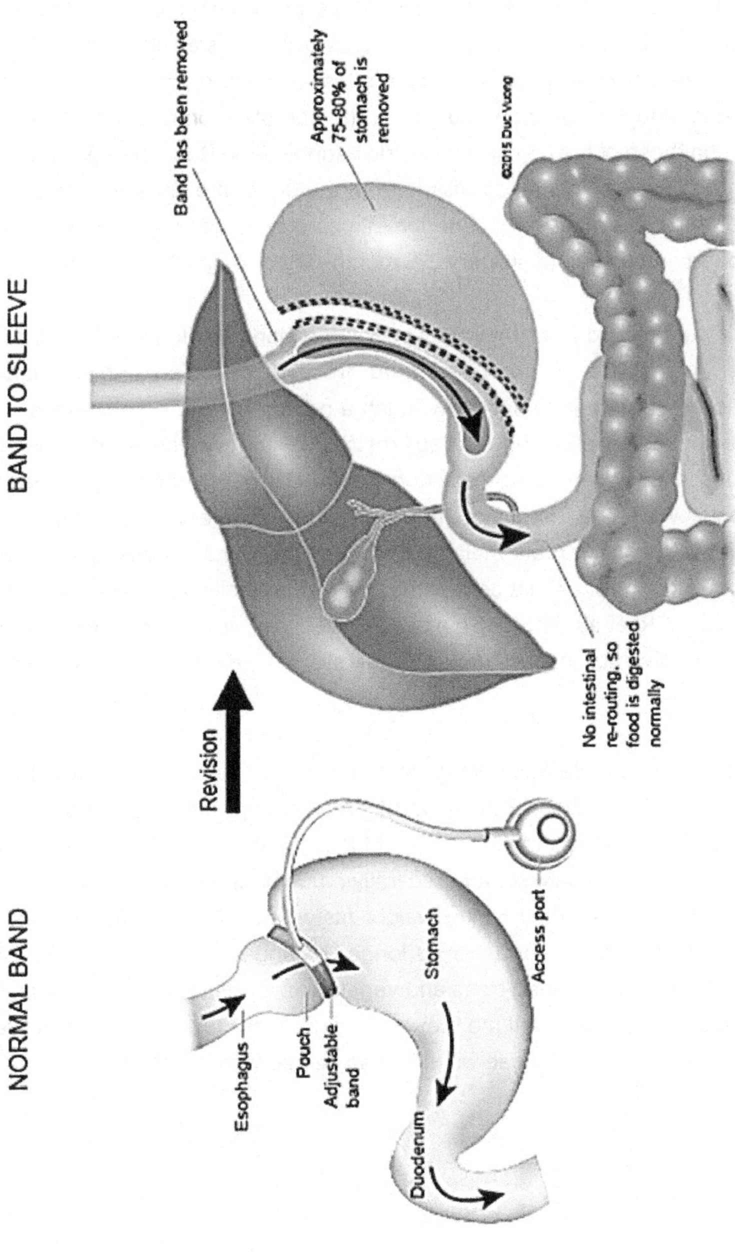

The vertical sleeve gastrectomy, often called simply the sleeve, removes approximately 75-80% of the stomach. The remaining stomach is a tubular pouch (resembling a hot dog or a jacket sleeve) that is less stretchy. **There is no mechanical device.** The new pouch holds a considerably smaller volume than the normal stomach, which reduces the amount of food that can be consumed. Short-term studies show that the sleeve is as effective as the Roux-en-Y gastric bypass in terms of weight loss and improvement or remission of diabetes, and is also a safer surgery. The complication rates of the sleeve fall between those of the adjustable gastric band and the Roux-en-y gastric bypass. If there is not too much scar tissue from the band, the revision can usually be performed in one surgery. But sometimes one surgery is needed to remove the band and a second surgery 3-6 months later completes the sleeve.

Some surgeons do not think that revising a band to sleeve is a good option since both surgeries are considered “restrictive.” The primary goal of a restrictive surgery is to limit how much a patient eats. So, to some, it doesn’t make sense to replace one “failed” restrictive surgery with another. However, revising a gastric band to a gastric sleeve is my favorite surgical option for patients. We are learning more and more about the sleeve every day, including that it has a considerable metabolic component, which means that the surgery affects gut hormones that control the body’s metabolism and effect on diabetes (Schauer, PR, et al., 2014.) So a band to sleeve revision is not simply replacing one restrictive surgery with more of the same—the sleeve is also a metabolic surgery.

Studies demonstrate that band to sleeve revisions result in good weight loss—sleeve revision patients are at least catching up with their primary sleeve counterparts in terms of excess weight loss. In my clinic, I see this every day. My band to sleeve patients are generally much happier than when they had the band: not only are they losing weight faster and more easily, they have an improved lifestyle. Foods are no longer getting stuck, they can eat a wider variety of foods including fruits and vegetables, and hunger is less of an issue. Overall, most patients tell me they never knew how they were able to live with the band, now that they see what life can be like with the sleeve.

Revise the Band to Roux-N-Y Gastric Bypass

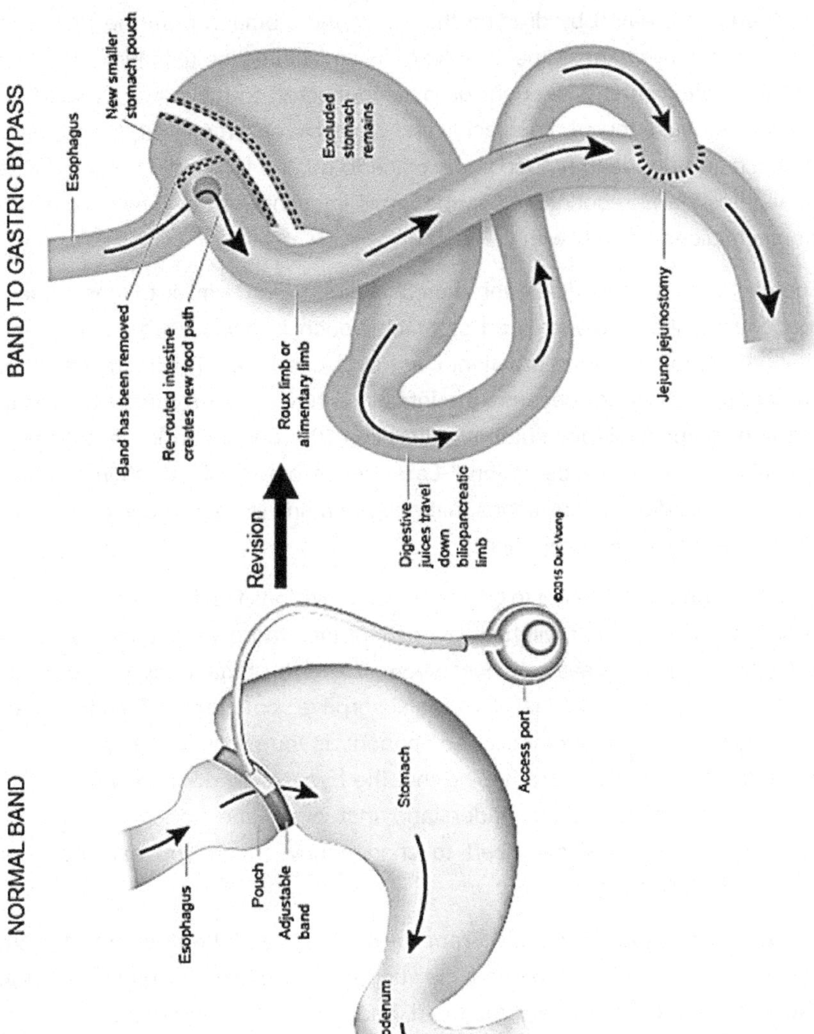

Most surgeons in the U.S. still consider the gastric bypass the Gold Standard of weight loss surgery, even though the sleeve surpassed the bypass as the most commonly performed bariatric surgery in 2013. I say "in the U.S." because this perception is quickly changing in the rest of the world. Major international bariatric societies think the sleeve will have become the number one weight loss surgery worldwide in 2015.

There are two components to the gastric bypass. First, a small stomach pouch, approximately one ounce in volume and about the size of a ping-pong ball or small egg, is created by dividing the top of the stomach from the rest of the stomach (the remnant stomach.) Next, the small intestine (jejunum) is divided, and the bottom end is brought up and connected to the newly created egg pouch. Because the stomach acids and digestive enzymes from the bypassed stomach and duodenum need some place to go, the top portion of the divided small intestine is reconnected to the small intestine further down so that the stomach juices can mix with the food.

The gastric bypass works by three mechanisms. First, similar to most bariatric procedures, the newly created stomach pouch is considerably smaller and limits the amount of food a patient can eat at one time. This is the restrictive component. Second, because the intestines have been rerouted to skip the segment responsible for nutrient absorption (the duodenum), the patient will experience some malabsorption. Last, the rerouting of digestion produces changes in endocrine hormones that reverse many illnesses such as diabetes. This is the metabolic component.

Surgeons who prefer band to gastric bypass revisions feel it adds a component of "malabsorption" that will help the patient lose more weight initially. Long-term, however, the gastric bypass seems to work primarily by the restrictive method. In other words, the malabsorptive component becomes less prominent, and the metabolic component is currently an active area of investigation. So if you are hoping that the bypass will do more work for you because of malabsorption, understand that over time you might lose that component. You will still need to change how much you eat and, more importantly, *what* you eat.

In this revision, the surgeon will remove the band and then perform a gastric bypass. As in the sleeve revision, the surgeon has to take down the scar tissue caused by the band, remove the band, and decide if it is safe to proceed with the bypass in the same surgery. If it is safe, then the surgeon must decide where to put the gastric pouch. Sometimes the pouch can be placed above or below where the band was, in which case it is called a micropouch. Some surgeons like to make longer, narrower pouches, so they might include the whole area of scar tissue that was taken down.

The shape and placement of the pouch are important to the patient's weight loss. They also dictate how and where the surgeon will connect your small intestine. This connection, called the GJ (gastrojejunal) anastamosis, is where most bypass leaks occur, so the tissue where it is created must be healthy. If it is not, the anastamosis is at a greater risk of leaking or coming apart. This leak will make the patient very ill and will most likely require an emergency surgery to fix. Most surgeons will place one or more drains after a band to bypass surgery and keep patients longer in the hospital to watch for leaks. This revision might require a stay in the ICU, but this depends on your surgeon's preferences and how the surgery went. Don't be upset if you wake up in the ICU—the surgeon is just taking extra precautions to keep you safe.

Bypass patients often get Dumping Syndrome, which occurs when a bypass patient eats something too sweet and the sugar load causes a fluid shift in the gut. This results in crampy abdominal pain, nausea, vomiting, and explosive diarrhea— a great deterrent to eating sweets. But not every bypass patient has dumping syndrome and most patients will lose this syndrome after a few years. I also see bypass patients who have dumping syndrome yet choose to have sweets and suffer the painful consequences.

My friend, Dr. Garth Davis from Houston, TX has much experience with revisional surgery and prefers to revise bands to RNY gastric bypass. He believes the band creates poor eating habits and that his band to bypass patients do very well because they can correct them. He says, "Just because a patient is not successful with a band does not mean she will not be successful with a bypass. My patients are much happier after revision to a bypass." I echo his sentiments that the band can create poor eating habits and also think a bypass is a very good option for revision.

Revise the Band to a Duodenal Switch

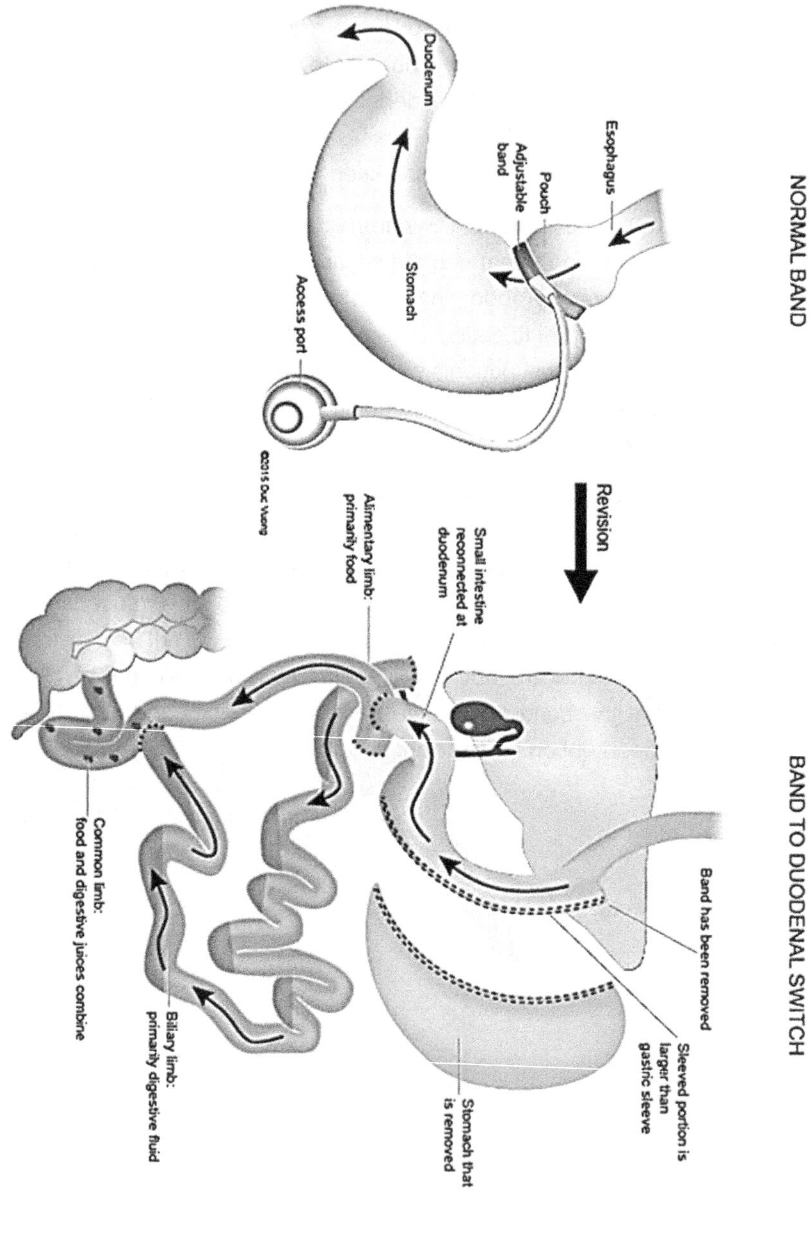

The Biliopancreatic Diversion with Duodenal Switch (BPD/DS), or Duodenal Switch (DS) for short, has two components. First a tubular stomach pouch (similar to the sleeve but about twice as large) is created by removing the stretchy portion of the stomach. Next, a large portion of the small intestine is bypassed. The duodenum is divided just past the outlet of the stomach. The last segment of the small intestine called the ileum is brought up and connected to the outlet of the newly created stomach. When the patient eats, the food goes through a newly created tubular stomach pouch and empties directly into the last segment of the small intestine, bypassing roughly three-fourths of the small intestine. The bypassed area, which carries the bile and pancreatic enzymes that are necessary for the breakdown and absorption of protein and fat, is reconnected to the last portion of the small intestine.

Similar to the other surgeries described above, the DS initially helps to reduce the amount of food that is consumed (it is restrictive); however, over time this effect lessens and patients are eventually able to consume nearly "normal" amounts of food. **Because the DS is extremely malabsorptive, the DS patient does need to eat larger portions than other weight-loss patients to get enough nutrition.** Of all weight loss procedures, the DS has the longest length of bypassed small bowel, meaning that the food does not mix with the digestive juices until very far down the gut and thus the patient does not absorb as many calories, nutrients, protein, and (most importantly for WLS patients) fat, including fat-soluble vitamins and nutrients. Lastly, the DS is also a metabolic surgery and probably has the best long-term improvement in illnesses such as diabetes. **But the trade-off is in the increased risk for other vitamin and nutritional problems like osteoporosis, hair loss, and chronic diarrhea.**

Here is how my colleague Dr. Nelson Trelles from France explains the DS as a revision:

> "Laparoscopic BPD-DS is performed in one or two steps, coupled with [removal] of the gallbladder. In experienced hands, postoperative complications are similar to a primary BPD-DS procedure (low morbidity and mortality). Frequent clinical and biological follow-up [...] is recommended as for any other bariatric procedure. Due to the sleeve gastrectomy component of the BPD-DS, patients rediscover more physiological and comfortable alimentary habits as compared to gastric band. Patients who do not wish to undergo the significant dietary or volume restrictions imposed by RYGB may opt for BPD-DS because of

> its substantially larger stomach pouch (150 – 200 mL). Previous gastric reflux usually associated with band is well controlled after BPD-DS. With the excellent outcomes obtained, patients regain confidence and improve quality of life. We obtain almost 100% resolution of Diabetes and most other comorbidities. Patients who require chronic high-dose anti-inflammatory medications (e.g., for severe arthritis) may also benefit from this less ulcerogenic procedure. Patients who require periodic surveillance of their stomach (e.g., Helicobacter pylori infection, chronic atrophic gastritis, ulcers, neoplasm and intestinal metaplasia) are also good candidates because the entire stomach remains accessible via upper endoscopy, contrary to RYGB. The most frequent concerns with this procedure are foul-smelling flatulence, diarrhea and malnutrition in the long-term. The first two symptoms can be effectively treated with dietary counseling or medications. Protein-enriched diets with twice-daily multivitamins (with iron and calcium supplements and fat-soluble vitamins: A, D, E and K) are recommended to prevent malnutrition and vitamin deficiencies."

As Dr. Trelles mentions above, with the malabsorptive power of the duodenal switch come some major trade-offs in lifestyle. One of the more limiting side-effects is multiple loose bowel movements, on average 4-7 a day. These bowel movements can be very fatty and foul-smelling, which might create embarrassing work or social situations. If the nature of your work means you don't have ready access to a bathroom—such as a police officer, chef, toll booth operator, or heart surgeon to name a few—then a DS might not be right for you. DS patients can also have an unusual body, sweat, or breath odor. While you might think these side-effects are trivial, patients have lost jobs and spouses because of them, so please consider this option carefully.

Revise the Band to Gastric Plication

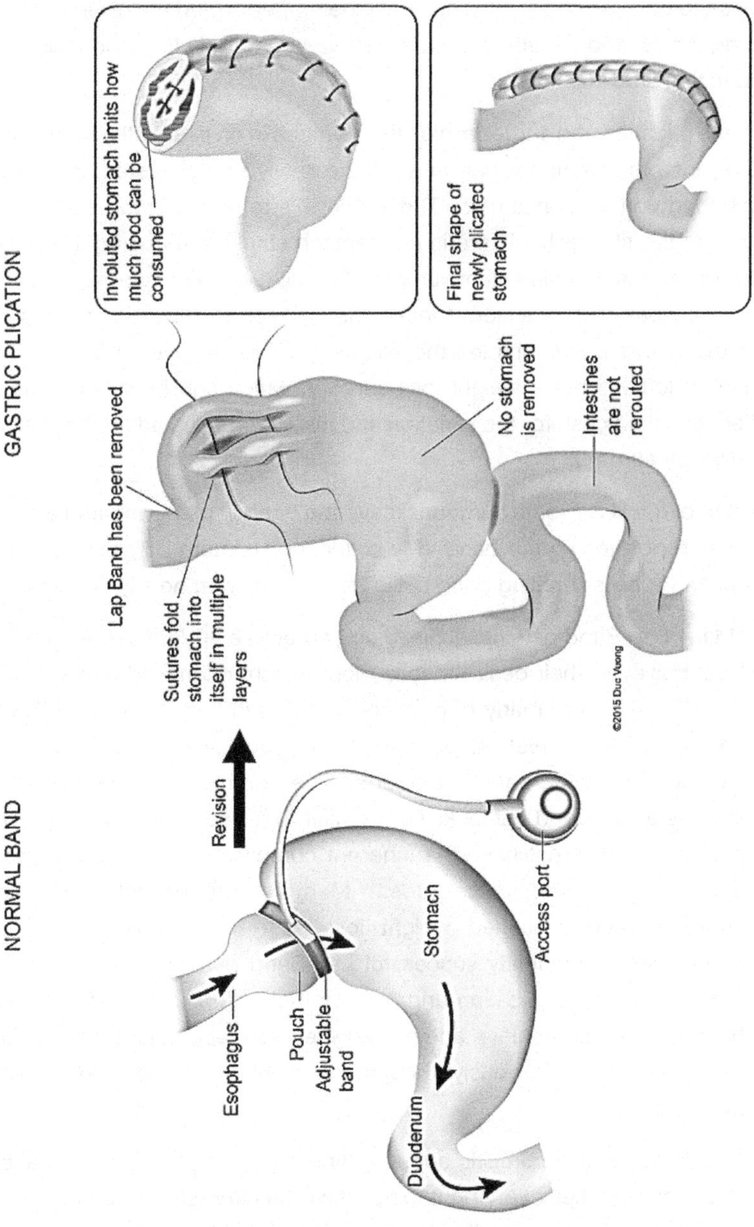

Greater curvature plication is a newer surgery that is still investigational in the U.S., meaning insurance will not currently cover it although some patients choose to pay cash for it. It is currently being performed mainly in Mexico, the Middle East, and South America, as well as in U.S. academic centers conducting studies.

With the plication, the surgeon folds the stomach in on itself with sutures, usually in 3 layers, but sometimes only in two. The newly involuted stomach limits how much food can be consumed. The concept is to replicate the sleeve without removing the stomach. There is no stomach stapling, reducing the likelihood of leaks. But leaks can still occur with the plication! Fixing a plication leak is technically easier than a sleeve leak—the surgeon takes you back to surgery, cuts the sutures, and unfolds the plication. This resolves the leak, but the patient is left without a weight loss surgery, which can be devastating if the patient has paid cash for the plication and now carries the additional cost of the emergency surgery.

Outside of the U.S., some surgeons leave the band in place and add a plication, possibly repositioning the band. My colleague Helmuth Billy has used this as an option for his struggling band patients. Here is what he says about it:

> "Many Lap-Band patients achieve an impressive 40-50% excess weight loss; however, their desire to lose more weight often leads them to ask "what next?" For many of my band patients in this quandary, I like to add a greater curvature plication to improve satiety by folding the stomach below the band into a tube. The end result is a stomach that still has a Lap-Band but looks very similar to a sleeve gastrectomy. The procedure does not have the inherent complications found with more aggressive stapling procedures. Many of my patients have had improved and sustained weight loss with this approach. In my experience, a modestly successful Lap-Band patient, who receives a greater curvature plication and renews their effort to maintain a good healthy diet, can achieve another 20% excess weight loss and sustain the result they previously thought was only possible with stapling procedures."

Dr. Billy is definitely optimistic about adding a gastric plication to a band, and with his results he has every right to be. It will be interesting to see if this option will be effective long-term. To clarify, adding a plication *without* removing the band is different than the photo above.

You might have read about getting a band AND plication during your initial weight loss surgery. This too is currently investigational and does not yet have long-term data. I discuss this more later.

Revise the Band to a Minigastric Bypass

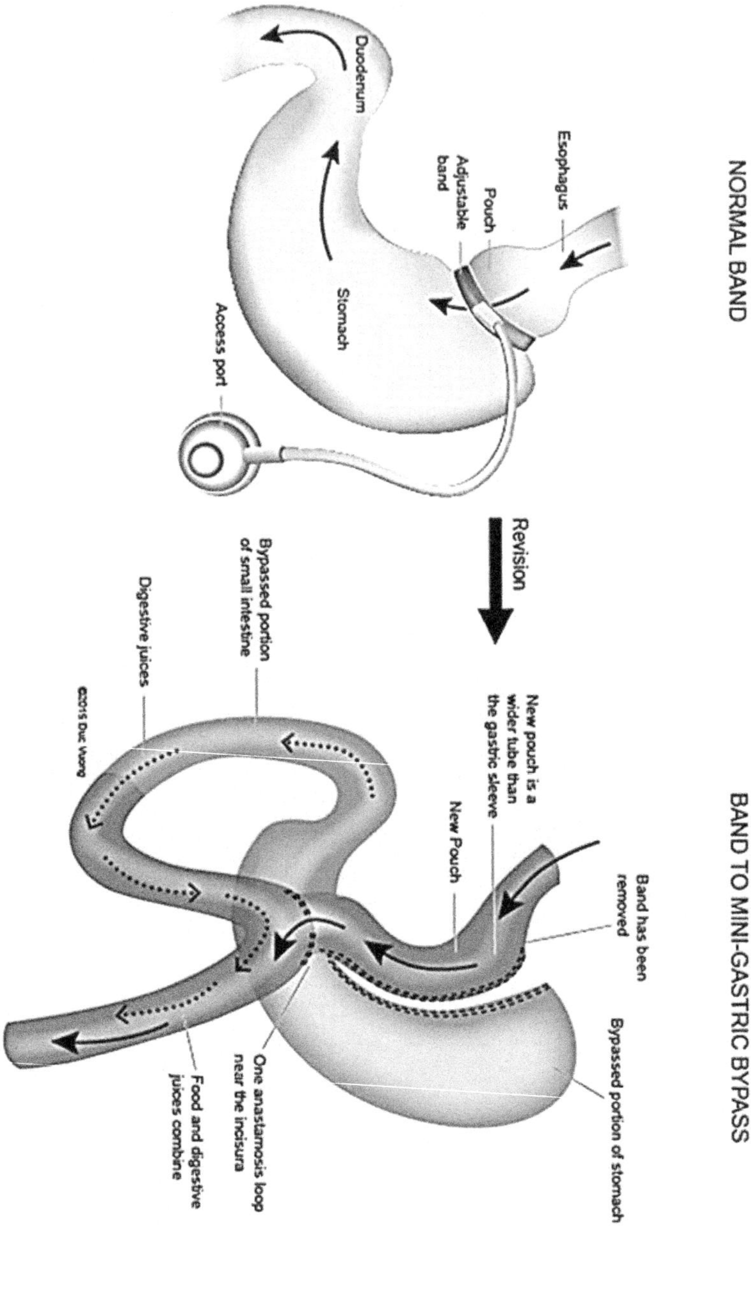

The Minigastric Bypass, also known as the One-Anastamosis Gastric Bypass, is becoming popular worldwide. It was pioneered by Dr. Robert Rutledge in Las Vegas, Nevada, but is currently not widely performed in the U.S., meaning once again that insurance will not cover it.

In the minigastric bypass, the surgeon makes a long, narrow pouch, similar to the sleeve but shorter. Unlike the sleeve, no portion of the stomach is removed. He then adds a single connection (anastamosis) between the small intestine and this pouch about 180-200cm down from the ligament of Treitz. It is possible that this way of connecting the small bowel has a larger malabsorptive component than the gastric bypass, but this is currently under debate. If this malabsorptive component is as powerful as it seems, surgeons are not sure if there will be increased risk of complications, although so far it appears to be safe and viable. My friend and colleague from Joplin, Missouri, Dr. David Hargoder, prefers the MGB, saying:

> "The minigastric bypass is an excellent choice to consider when faced with Lap-Band failure. The removal of the Lap-Band and conversion to a MGB can be performed in about an hour with an overnight stay in the hospital. Adding the malabsorptive component, which the MGB provides, produces immediate results when weight loss stalls after the restrictive-only Lap-Band. The technical simplicity of the MGB along with its excellent weight loss results [and] outstanding safety profile, and the ability to reverse or revise the MGB easily if necessary, makes it the preferred option in my practice."

Do not be misled by the name "mini" gastric bypass. This is a major surgery with major considerations! Since its pouch is similar to the sleeve, you will have the same considerations as revising to the sleeve, but in addition you will have an anastamosis to contend with. This anastamosis could leak, twist, kink, or cause bile reflux, which is different from acid reflux. Some surgeons are concerned that this exposure to bile might lead to an increased risk of gastric cancer, but to date, no studies have confirmed this suspicion. There are also not too many surgeons currently performing this procedure in America, so you might be limited in access.

Robotic Surgery

Robotic surgery refers not to a surgery itself but to a different access platform by which the surgeon can perform all of the above surgeries. There are some definite advantages to having your revisional surgery performed robotically. My friend, Dr. Tomasz Rogula from the Cleveland Clinic, explains it like this:

> "I prefer the robotic approach because it makes the surgery much easier. I believe that the dissection of the tissues is much clearer. I also prefer it for the handsewn gastrojejunal anastamosis, which is a critical step in a bypass surgery."

Most surgeons agree that the 3-D optics and refined motions achievable with the robot are currently superior to standard laparoscopy. The debate continues, however, over whether or not these technical benefits of robotic technology will justify the significant increase in cost.

In Summary

Revisional surgery has increased risks, so don't make your decision lightly. A lot depends on where you live, the access you have to medical care, and the surgeon you choose. If you came to see me, I would probably recommend a revision to a sleeve, which your insurance would most likely cover; but if you went to see Dr. Hargroder in Missouri, you would probably get a mini-gastric bypass and pay cash. Dr. Hargroder is an excellent surgeon who is as passionate about the minigastric bypass as I am about the sleeve. Every surgeon has a preference in revisional surgery, so make sure you discuss his reasons for recommending a particular surgery to you and share your informed concerns with him.

Regardless of which procedure you choose, you will still need to change your diet and lifestyle. No revisional surgery will work otherwise.

Surgery	Advantages	Disadvantages
Reband	▪ No anemia ▪ No dumping ▪ No malabsorption ▪ Very low mortality rate ▪ Adjustability ▪ Removable ▪ Laparoscopic revision ▪ Leaves opportunities for future revisions or interventions.	▪ Purely restrictive ▪ Band could reslip ▪ Band or tubing leakage ▪ Port Infection ▪ Band Infection ▪ Regurgitation due to esophageal obstruction ▪ Band erosion into the stomach ▪ Esophageal dilatation ▪

Sleeve	▪ Restrictive ▪ Considered a metabolic surgery ▪ Weight loss similar to that of the gastric bypass at 3-5 years ▪ Probably a lower complication rate than gastric bypass ▪ No foreign device ▪ No intestinal re-routing ▪ Leaves opportunities for future revisions or interventions.	▪ Is "non-reversible," though the sleeve could stretch out ▪ Leaks can be difficult to heal or fix ▪ The staple line of the sleeve might go directly over the scar tissue from the band ▪ Surgeon might need to make a larger sleeve than usual due to scar tissue at the GEJ. ▪
RNY Gastric Bypass	▪ Mostly restrictive ▪ Some malabsorption ▪ Metabolic surgery ▪ Typical maintenance of >60% excess weight loss long-term	▪ Technically complex with higher complication rates ▪ Possible long-term vitamin/mineral deficiencies ▪ Potential for dumping syndrome ▪ Requires adherence to dietary recommendations, life-long vitamin/mineral supplementation, and follow-up compliance
Duodenal Switch	▪ Probably greater weight loss than RYGB, LSG, or AGB ▪ The most metabolic surgery ▪ Patients eventually eat nearly "normal-sized" meals ▪ Reduces the absorption of fat by 70 percent or more ▪ Is the most effective against diabetes	▪ Highest complication rates and risk of mortality ▪ Greatest risk of protein deficiencies and long-term deficiencies in many vitamins and minerals ▪ Compliance with follow-up visits and strict adherence to dietary and vitamin supplementation guidelines are critical ▪ Diarrhea on average of 4-7 times a day

	compared to RYGB, LSG, and AGB	▪ Frequent passing of foul-smelling gas ▪ Changes in body odor ▪ Gas pains or bloating ▪ Hair loss
Plication	▪ No rerouting of intestines ▪ No implantation of a banding device ▪ Could be performed without removing the band ▪ Reversible	▪ Purely restrictive ▪ Newer procedure with unproven long-term effectiveness ▪ Not covered by insurance ▪ Possible separation of sutured areas ▪ Possible obstruction of lumen (food cannot pass through) ▪ Leaks from sutured areas
Minigastric Bypass	▪ Restrictive and malabsorptive ▪ Long-term weight loss of 75-80% ▪ Low rate of complications ▪ Bypassed intestine can be easily lengthened if inadequate weight loss ▪ Reversible	▪ Still investigational ▪ Not covered by insurance ▪ Risk of leaks ▪ Bile reflux ▪ Nutrient malabsorption ▪ Limited access to the surgery

Summary and Tips: "Which surgery is the RIGHT CHOICE for me?"

1) Revisional surgery has increased risk of complications, so you must be clear on why you want another surgery. Write down your reasons for wanting to be revised.

____

____

____

____

2) Each surgery has its pro's and con's. Based on the above information, which surgery appeals to you most and why?

____

____

____

____

3) Do an internet search on that procedure. Watch YouTube videos. Avoid "patient testimonial" type of websites or videos.

4) Call your bariatric surgeon to see if he offers revisional surgery and if so, then ask which procedures he offers.

11

Playing The Insurance Game

"You have to learn the rules of the game. And then you have to play better than anyone else." *– Albert Einstein*

"Will my insurance cover another surgery?" is a simple question with a complicated answer. The short version is "Yes, usually, maybe, but it depends..." Here are a few issues that affect the answer:

1. Does your insurance policy allow revision or is there an exclusion or a "one surgery per lifetime" maximum?
2. Do you have the same insurance that covered your original band surgery?
3. Did you pay cash for your band, which means your current insurance might consider your condition a "pre-existing illness"?
4. What is your current BMI? Is it too low to meet criteria?
5. Do you have symptoms or complications other than weight regain, like abdominal pain, difficulty swallowing, reflux, or recurrent pneumonia?
6. Does your surgeon even do revisions? If so, will he do a revision on you?

My clinic has been fortunate in that we have not had many problems with getting revisional bariatric surgery covered in New Mexico, but this could change at any time. For us, getting revisional surgery approved usually just involves submitting the requisite paperwork for preapproval to the insurance company. Our program, however, has additional requirements in order to consider revisions, assuming that it is not an emergency situation. I deflate the band completely for three months with monthly dietary visits, during which the patient *must* demonstrate weight loss through adherence to proper nutritional choices. In addition, the patient attends my Patient Empowerment Program (PEP), which is a weekly series of educational groups that I personally lead. We get to know patients very well, and if any single member of our bariatric team (including my office manager, dietitians, medical assistant, and front office staff) has concerns about the patient, the patient's surgery will be reviewed, discussed and possibly delayed. All of this helps bolster our case to insurance companies for coverage. As I've mentioned earlier, I currently believe that a band to sleeve revision has acceptable risks for considerable reward, but of course, this might change depending on long-term results.

American military insurance has a distinct set of limitations. The U.S. military requires that surgeons try to find one weight loss surgery that best suits the patient. It is my understanding that revisional surgery is scrutinized very closely in the military, but I do not have personal experience with this. As of the writing of this book, Tricare, the military insurance company, covers either the band or the gastric bypass, so even if they approve a revision, you will be limited to the gastric bypass as your only choice.

If you live in a country with socialized medicine, such as Canada or England, you might face major hurdles. England, for example, requires that the surgeon appeal to the government for approval of revisional surgery, a long process with a low success rate. I'm not an expert on socialized medicine, so it would be best to contact your local surgeon in countries with that system. Here is what my colleague, Cynthia-Michelle Borg, MD FRCS, at University Hospital Lewisham in London, says about revisional surgery in the UK:

> "The most recent UK National Bariatric Surgery Registry (NBSR) report indicated that about 7% of bariatric procedures performed between 2011 and 2013 were revisional procedures. Currently, the National Health Service (NHS) in England only funds revisions
>
> 1) in patients who develop a complication related to their original operation like slippage or erosion associated with gastric band, severe reflux after sleeve gastrectomy or stricture/nutritional problems after gastric bypass or duodenal switch surgery. Conversion to another bariatric procedure is funded if clinically indicated.
>
> 2) when a two-staged procedure is indicated, e.g. in super-morbidly obese patients.
>
> Patients who have not reached their expected weight loss targets or who have regained weight after the primary operation are not routinely funded. This includes patients with a dilated gastric pouch or dilated gastro-jejunal anastomosis post-gastric bypass. If there are exceptional clinical circumstances, an application to the regional Individual Funding Request panel can be made by the treating clinicians (however, such requests are frequently rejected).
>
> These strict criteria may lead patients to seek revisional surgery in the private sector or outside the UK. Patients looking into this option need to do their research carefully regarding the surgeon's experience and the clinic's facilities. They also need to be sure what is included in the package, as these operations tend to be more difficult and are associated with higher complication rates and costs compared to primary operations."

Common Insurance Scenarios

Here are a few possible scenarios in which gastric band patients might find themselves:

1) "My surgeon retired and I can't find anyone willing to provide care for me."—Whether your surgeon retired or moved away, or you moved to a new region, you are now in search of a new healthcare provider who is knowledgeable about gastric bands. Hopefully, your surgeon made arrangements for you to see a different surgeon, but that doesn't always happen. I've heard some scenarios in which surgeons in the same city will not see a patient from one of their competitors. To me, such competition seems arbitrary and punishes the patient, and I try to accept or help any patients in need. The best way to contact me if you need help in the New Mexico area is to visit our website at www.LovelaceBariatrics.com. Some Lap-Band fill centers will accept new band patients, but unfortunately many of them have gone out of business.

2) "I lost my insurance," or "My insurance no longer covers bariatric surgery."—I've seen this scenario too many times to count. People change jobs and companies change insurance policies, often annually, sometimes as a cost-saving measure. Maybe your insurance was through your spouse's company, and now they've changed policies or he has lost his job. Don't give up—you can find a new carrier that does cover bariatrics or pay the cash price for a visit with a qualified bariatric surgeon. Taking these steps is well worth it, given the possible cost of a complication or the risk of permanent damage to your body.

3) "I had my surgery out of the country and cannot find anyone willing to take care of me."—In my practice, we always adopt patients who have had surgery elsewhere because our purpose is to provide a service to the community, not to punish patients for taking steps to better their lives. Unfortunately, not every surgeon or practice feels the same way, so be wary when out-of-the-country clinics promise, "You can just follow up with your primary care doctor." Many surgeons do not want to take on the liability of a complication from another surgeon, especially when the surgery was performed in a different country.

4) "My BMI is below 30 so I don't qualify for a revisional surgery, but I'm struggling!"—This is a common scenario, too. With hard work and determination, you've managed to get your BMI below 30, but still not to your goal. Then something happens, like a band slip. Your surgeon recommends leaving your band deflated since there is no emergency, but maybe you'd like a revisional surgery. You learn, however, that you no longer qualify for weight loss surgery due to your low BMI. While this seems unfair, doctors need to follow existing medical guidelines in addition to guidelines set forth by insurance policies.

"I HOPE YOU WILL TAKE THIS OPPORTUNITY TO VIEW THE BAND AS HAVING BEEN SUCCESSFUL."

> It got the weight off and maybe got you off some medicines. Hopefully you've taken this time to change your dietary habits and figure out some issues that were keeping you from being healthy. Instead of being frustrated by insurance, the program, or the surgeon, view this as an opportunity to use what you've learned to stay successful.

Some frustrated band patients who are suffering with symptoms such as nausea, vomiting, dehydration, or abdominal pain, decide to go to the local emergency room for treatment. They are usually disappointed by the results of this ER visit, which may provide the patients with some IV fluids, medications to help control their symptoms, blood work, and a CT scan, which usually returns as normal. The patients are then discharged home to "follow-up with their surgeons." But these problems occurred because the patients do not have surgeons to see in the first place! Unfortunately, in many communities, emergency rooms are not equipped to care for weight loss surgery patients properly, due to lack of resources, education, or availability of a bariatric surgeon. So patients, though maybe feeling a little relief from the pain and anti-nausea medicines, are still in their original quandary. **Don't assume that going to the emergency room will solve your problems—the ER physician can only provide you with the resources available to him.** These ER visits, while relevant to the patient, may have little or no bearing on your insurance's coverage of a revision.

Based on the urgency of your symptoms, some surgeons might perform a revision under a different diagnosis code from the one likely used for your original surgery, 278.01 Morbid Obesity. Insurance coverage depends on the diagnosis code associated with the need for a procedure. For example, if you need to have your appendix removed, the diagnosis code would be 540.9 Appendicitis, which could then be furthered qualified as acute, perforated, etc. Depending on your symptoms and the status of your band and surrounding areas, a surgeon could use an *appropriate* code different from Morbid Obesity to remove your band, and possibly even revise you to a different surgery. This is situation- and surgeon-dependent.

Like all ethical surgeons, I always follow proper coding guidelines, but I also focus on the educational component of the surgery. Even if a band patient has an appropriate code other than Morbid Obesity, I insist that the patient go through my educational process (unless it is an emergency surgery). A few patients have chosen to go to other programs with less stringent education requirements, but I believe that **education is the key to weight loss surgery success.** Even if your insurance will cover revisional surgery, remember that all weight loss surgeries have their pro's and con's. Avoid thinking, "Everything would be fixed if I could only get a new surgery." You have to change your behaviors, and that starts by changing your thinking. Have a serious heart-to-heart talk with that person in the mirror, because...

"REVISIONAL BARIATRIC SURGERY ENTAILS SIGNIFICANTLY INCREASED RISK OF COMPLICATIONS, ADDITIONAL MEDICAL COSTS, AND UNKNOWN LONG-TERM SUCCESS RATES."

Because of a lack of good data, surgeons do not have a consensus on which revisional procedures are best, much less which patients should receive them. If you think everything will be better if your insurance would only approve your next surgery, there will most likely be another and then another surgery in your life.

Summary and Tips: "Am I prepared for an insurance BATTLE?"

1) Insurance plans vary in their coverage of revisional surgery. I recommend that you do not call the company yourself but rather let your bariatric surgeon's office call on your behalf.

2) Do you know your BMI? Use an online BMI calculator to make sure your BMI is still within most insurance guidelines for bariatric coverage (BMI ≥ 40 or BMI ≥ 35 with a comorbidity.) If your BMI is between 35-40, then you will need an accompanying illness, such as diabetes, hypertension, arthritis, or sleep apnea to qualify.

3) Are you having complications from your band, such as a dilated esophagus, band slippage, or aspiration? These complications might help bolster your case for a revision.

4) Have you asked your coworker how she got her revision covered?

5) Do you have the financial resources to pay cash for a revision? Have you looked into more affordable, yet reputable options outside of your country?

12

The Future of the Gastric Band

"The report of my death was an exaggeration." *– Mark Twain, American author, upon reading a news item that he was ill and possibly dying.*

In Fall 2013, news that Allergan had sold their division responsible for manufacturing the Lap-Band to the smaller company Apollo Endosurgery, set the bariatric community abuzz. Most surgeons, especially the ones who still believed in the efficacy of the band, applauded the sale as a good move for bariatric surgery. After all, Apollo Endosurgery specializes in developing new surgical product lines, while Allergan is a conglomerate of diverse divisions and products. Enthusiastic surgeons believed the Lap-Band would finally get the attention it deserved as a weight loss surgery option and hoped that Apollo would invest in the development of new band technologies, such as a self-adjusting port.

Here is a statement for this book from Mr. Michael Oberg, the senior director of marketing for Apollo Endosurgery, regarding the future of the Lap-Band:

> "Apollo Endosurgery is excited about the future of weight loss surgery and is committed to addressing the obesity epidemic by increasing access to care and innovating with new products. The LAP-BAND System has a bright future ahead and will continue to be a viable option for obese patients who are looking to combat their weight issues. As the only FDA-approved device for patients with a BMI of at least 30 with one obesity related condition, the LAP-BAND System should also be considered for lower BMI patients as a preventative to severe obesity and its health consequences. We look forward to evolving the LAP-BAND into more than just a weight-loss procedure, but into a full solution that patients can rely on for strength and support throughout their weight loss journey."

Apollo is clearly bullish on the band, but it has many possible futures:

New bands—Will Apollo invest in developing a new band, much like Allergan did in 2008 with the AP Band? The AP Band was a major improvement over earlier bands and is still in use today. The AP band is wider with a better balloon intended to provide more concentric and uniform compression around the stomach. The AP band is also easier to unbuckle than the old band, making placement and revisions simpler. Surgeons no longer struggle to unbuckle or cut the band, leaving the option to reuse or reposition it in cases of band slips.

At the time of writing, Apollo Endosurgery has not disclosed plans for any updates to the design of the Lap-Band. Given the current downward trend in band placements worldwide, Apollo may not see rejuvenation of the band as cost-effective.

Self-adjusting ports—Can you imagine a band that self-adjusts? Imagine a band that is looser in the mornings, when band patients complain about sliming and restriction, but tighter during the day when mindless grazing is more of an issue. All of this would be automatic without the need for any needle sticks. This technology was in development a few years ago, but the research was shelved. The hope was that the band could sense the appropriate amount of restriction needed at various times for the patient to be successful and comfortable. It is too early to tell if Apollo will reinvest in this technology, but many band surgeons hope they will. And I'm sure many patients would welcome such an innovation!

Banded plication—Some surgeons think that a band placed at the same time as a gastric plication is a better than a band alone. This approach is being performed mostly outside of the United States or under investigational review boards (IRBs) in the United States, so it is not widely available to patients. To clarify, this is a surgery in which the band is placed at the *same* time as the gastric plication, and is distinct from a plication that is added to a band as a revision surgery. Why band a plication? Data suggest that banded plication has better initial weight loss than plication alone, so at least for the next few years, the band will be around as a part of this developing procedure. Apollo may investigate new band variations that make it more effective in combination with the plication (or as part of the two surgeries below).

Banded sleeve—A few surgeons place bands around patients who have regained weight after a gastric sleeve. Some surgeons place a band at the same time as they perform the sleeve with acceptable short-term outcomes. I'm not sure of the long-term efficacy of either procedure, but it will be exciting to see how this surgery affects patients' bodies and mindsets during their weight loss journey. Such procedures are performed primarily outside of the United States, so again access might be an issue.

Banded bypass—The procedure with the most data is the banded bypass. This is a RNY gastric bypass with a band placed above the GJ anastamosis (where the small intestine is connected to the new egg-sized stomach pouch) in one surgery. **This is NOT the same as a band that is placed on a failed or struggling bypass!** With an adjustable gastric band around the bypass pouch, the patient can receive adjustments postoperatively as needed to keep the jejunum immediately below the GJ anastamosis from stretching and creating a new food reservoir. The band could also keep the pouch from dilating. Dr. Mathias Fobi is the pioneer for this procedure and probably has the most extensive experience with it. He has published data that suggest that the banded bypass has better long-term outcomes than regular RNY bypass and has developed his own version of the band. When asked for a quote for this book, Dr. Fobi commented,

> "Pouch dilation is part of the natural history of any operation for obesity that has restriction as one of its mechanisms for effectiveness. Placing a ring or band around the pouch leaving a small pouch, smaller than 30 cc, enhances the weight loss and weight loss maintenance after such an operation."

Some surgeons worldwide will put in a non-adjustable band at the time of a gastric bypass. This is not the same as putting in an adjustable band (Lap-Band.)

Even though these procedures are probably not options for your case, the gastric band will likely continue to be available in different forms and procedures. So the death of the band is not as close as some might lead you to think.

Summary and Tips: "I might want to WAIT and SEE what happens."

1) Apollo has started a new advertising campaign for the band. Currently the Lap-band is the only FDA-approved weight loss surgery for patients with BMI between 30-35. If you have a low BMI, a new band model might be an option for you, especially if you had your band placed prior to 2008.

2) There are newer options on the horizon, such as intragastric balloons and duodenal endobarrier. Do you want to wait for these new technologies evolve?

13

"I'm Struggling, What Should I Do Now?"

***"Strength does not come from winning. Your struggles develop your strengths. When you go through hardships and decide not to surrender, that is strength."** – Arnold Schwarzenegger*

Maybe you are not quite ready to give up on your band, maybe you are without insurance coverage, or maybe your life circumstances are keeping you from following through with another surgery. Maybe you're not sure if you can handle another surgery emotionally or want to go through a new set of side effects. But if you are inspired to get back on track, here are a few suggestions about what you might do now to help clarify the picture.

Check with your bariatric surgeon. Get to your surgeon's office right away. Do not wait until the 10 pounds you have regained become 30 pounds and the 30 pounds become 50 pounds. Your surgeon will need to assess whether or not something is wrong with your gastric band, like a pouch dilatation that has allowed you to eat more than you should. Many patients wait too long to return to the surgeon, and as a consequence, develop severe damage to their esophagus or upper stomach.

When you go back to a surgeon, make sure you see a bariatric surgeon, preferably the one who did your surgery. A general surgeon might not have the expertise to understand band-related difficulties or complications, and most primary care doctors will not have enough expertise to correctly diagnose and treat your weight regain. Likewise, I would not recommend a "fill center" or a non-surgeon physician who provides band adjustments. While these places and providers are helpful with routine maintenance care, if you are struggling with your band, you need more expertise: **You need an experienced bariatric surgeon**.

Do not let distance or inconvenience deter you from getting the help you need. One time my clinic received a phone call from a Band patient who could not swallow anything and was in a rural hospital three hours away. She kept telling the doctors there that her band needed to be deflated. Their response was that they did not know how to do that, so they were going to perform open surgery to remove the band. She left AMA (against medical advice) and came to my clinic the next morning. I deflated her, and she immediately felt better. Imagine the consequences if she had not had the knowledge, courage, or gumption to call my office!

Consider a total unfill, going on a liquid diet, and re-starting. Every two years, I recommend what I call a "Lap-Band Vacation." I discussed this earlier. We all need regular vacations in our lives to release some of the stress of daily living, and your esophagus needs a break from working constantly against the band. The Lap-Band Vacation starts with an office visit and check-up, a complete dietary review, and a barium swallow to assess the position of your band and the appearance of your esophagus and upper stomach. I then schedule an EGD to visualize the appearance of the esophageal tissues and the pouch as well as to make sure the band has not eroded. I also watch in real time as your esophagus contracts and works—this gives me a good idea of how "tired" or "sluggish" it is, or, in other words, how badly it needs a vacation! If it seems to be working too hard or inefficiently, I completely deflate the band and place the patient on a minimum of two weeks of Optifast and fresh juices, which offer good nutrition. Blended smoothies with fresh fruits, vegetables, and tofu provide complete nutrition and are much healthier than packaged protein shakes or drinks. I do not have any studies or data to prove that this Lap-Band Vacation works to improve esophageal functioning, but my patients tell me that they feel better after a band vacation—partly because it "feels better" but mostly because it gets them back on track with weight loss.

"But how is this different from when my band slipped and my doctor deflated my band and restricted me to liquids for two weeks?" you ask. In a band slip scenario, the deflation is *not* a welcomed event, but rather usually viewed as a "failure" or "hassle." With the Lap-Band Vacation, it is planned and embraced. It is routine maintenance to keep your band working well, while the slip scenario is more like having your car break down on the freeway during morning rush hour traffic! Often during unexpected deflations, patients will "splurge" and gain weight. They might think, "I can finally eat!" and not make the best food choices. During a Band Vacation, patients are expected to lose weight by making healthy choices such as juicing fruits and vegetables and eating tofu. They revisit the Three Rules that we teach in our clinic, discussed below. I also cover these rules in more detail in *Ultimate Gastric Sleeve Success.*

Revise what you eat through volumetric eating. Nutritionist Barbara Rolls, PhD, created the principles behind volumetric eating in her 2000 book, *The Volumetrics Weight-Control Plan*. Her approach is to eat foods high in volume but low in calories, focusing on the feeling of fullness rather than food type. Rolls says that people feel full because of the amount of food they eat, not because of the number of calories or the grams of fat, protein, or carbohydrates in that food. This is similar to my approach. Here are the Three Rules my patients follow:

Rule #1: Lean protein comes first.

Rule #2: Fill your pouch with the most nutritious food you can most of the time.

Rule #3: You can eat all of the fresh fruits and vegetables you want, as much as you want, whenever you want.

You should focus on filling your pouch with nutritious foods. Not doing so greatly contributes to weight regain. If you cannot eat fresh fruits and vegetables, ask to be deflated slightly so that you can eat them comfortably. More importantly, these Rules apply regardless of which surgery you've had or are thinking of having. A brief explanation of these Rules is in Appendix B.

Reassess your choices. Barring any catastrophe with your band, the reason people regain weight after weight loss surgery is the same reason they become overweight in the first place—**consistently poor food choices**. Whether or not you want to admit this to your surgeon, you must admit it to yourself. You might feel like you have legitimate reasons for making poor food choices—your mother is sick, you're going through a divorce, you lost your job, your dog just died—but at the end of the day, eating poorly will not make you feel better about what happened.

- Your mother is the one with the illness, so you will need good food in order to have the energy to care for her.
- If you were in an unhappy marriage, a divorce should be a relief, not a stressor. You will need real food in order to have the energy to focus on the legal proceedings.
- If your company down-sized, you will need energy in order to find another, better job.

These are not reasons to give up all of the hard work you put into your weight loss journey. Don't settle for the label of a "stress eater" or "emotional eater," and instead figure out why you make the food choices you do during stressful times.

Start food journaling to find areas for improvement. A revision patient admitted recently that she was grazing on snacks of chips, candy, and crackers all day long, but was surprised that she had gained back 80 of the 130 pounds she had lost. The weight gain had very little to do with her new infant or boyfriend's bad influence. Why would you subject yourself to another surgery, when you could just change your food choices? I had a patient tell me once, "But Dr. Vuong, if I could eat fruits and vegetables, then I wouldn't need the surgery!" This is the same poor thinking that led her to become obese in the first place, and the same thinking that made her stall and regain with the Band.

Let go of the idea that a weight loss surgery, *any* weight loss surgery, will FORCE you to make better food choices.

You control your life; your mind is too powerful to be limited by any surgery or scheme, as in the example of that patient who continued to eat sweets despite terrible dumping syndrome. Surgery, especially revisional surgery, is a serious decision, so take the time to delve into deeper issues. Take a closer look at why you do the things you do, why you react the way you react, and why you think the way you think.

Get back to group. The best way to be successful is to surround yourself with successful people. That is true for all aspects of life, and so it is true for weight loss surgery. If you are struggling with your surgery, get back into a support group, preferably one that is well-run and monitored. If your surgeon does not have one, there are many other options. Find one led by a healthcare professional and not by well-meaning patients. You can also try established groups like Overeaters Anonymous, Weight Watchers, or medical weight loss programs, like an Optifast Meal Replacement Program, to get you back on track.

Sometimes patients say, "I'm too far from my surgeon for regular visits or support groups. I drive 4 hours round trip for a 2 minute visit to be told, 'It looks like you're doing fine.'" While not every surgeon is as engaged in support groups as I am, I can say that every surgeon wants patients to attend support group and tries hard to make sure they are convenient.

You can try internet groups such as ObesityHelp.com or BariatricPal.com (formerly LapBandTalk.com). There are also groups on Facebook. Keep in mind, however, that everybody has different experiences, some of these Internet groups are not carefully monitored, and patients—well-meaning as they may be—are not qualified to give medical advice. (You shouldn't be seeking medical advice on the Internet in the first place!) Some people feel bold behind the anonymity of the World Wide Web and make inappropriate or inaccurate statements.

You can join my secret Facebook sleeve group. Just friend me and ask to be added to the "secret group."

"TO FRIEND ME ON FACEBOOK, SEARCH FOR 'DUC VUONG' AND LOOK FOR THE DIRECTOR OF LOVELACE BARIATRICS. THEN ASK TO BE ADDED TO THE SECRET GROUP."

You can also find a good book to read on the subject. My other book, *Ultimate Gastric Sleeve Success*, addresses how to break a weight loss plateau or reverse weight regain. *Weight Loss Surgery Success: Dr. V's A-Z Steps on Losing Weight and Gaining Enlightenment* provides psychological and self-improvement tips beyond the usual "dieting" advice. And of course there are other books by other authors that could provide just the help you need.

Technology is making it ever easier to stay connected. Live streaming video platforms like Periscope and Meerkat allow patients in interact with healthcare providers instantly. **You can chat with me live on my nightly Periscope broadcast called "Real Talk With Dr. V" by following me @DrDucVuong.** Just download the Periscope app on your smart phone to get started.

Give yourself some credit. Stop letting the scale be your judge and jury. Remember the long-term average Excess Weight Loss Percentage (EWL%) with the Lap-Band is about 40%. This means if you are 100 pounds overweight, then you would likely keep off about 40 pounds at 5 years after the surgery. So if you are 5'4" tall and weigh 240 pounds, you will most likely weigh 200 pounds after 5 years. If you are doing better than 40% EWL (even if you are having problems with your band), you have above average results! Pounds lost are only one measure of success. Think about how much better you feel, how much more energy you have, how much further you can walk without getting short of breath. Be thankful if you have been able to decrease a few medicines, your blood sugars are better controlled, or you're off your CPAP machine. These are all wonderful milestones, so give yourself some credit.

Go to patient conferences. There are some great conferences put on by passionate advocates. Check out the Weight Loss Surgery Foundation of America (WLSFA), the Obesity Action Coalition (OAC), or the Texas Association for Bariatric Surgery (TABS), to name a few examples. Such conferences host talks and discussions with doctors and other medical professionals, and I'm often an invited speaker at these conferences, so maybe I will meet you at one someday. Some are in fun locations like Las Vegas or on a cruise ship, so you can really make an experience out of them!

Check with your insurance for revisional coverage. Many companies will cover revisions without making you repeat all of the initial requirements, but that can vary. Lack of insurance coverage, however, is not a reason not to see your surgeon. Often his office can tell you if a revisional surgery will be covered and, if not, offer alternatives. Revisional bariatric surgery coverage can be complicated and varies from state to state. Let the experts help you with the final insurance coverage, but get the ball rolling by understanding your insurance plan better. If you know a coworker with your same insurance coverage who has had revisional bariatric surgery, ask her what she had to do to get the surgery covered. The answer might be as simple as, "I just called my surgeon's office, and they took care of the rest!"

The point is that you don't need to "wait and see." **Take action now by asking questions and doing some research.**

Summary and Tips: "How can I get BACK ON TRACK?"

1) Call your surgeon's office now. Ask to make an appointment to have your Lap-Band evaluated and discuss revision options.

"My next appointment with my surgeon is ______________________________."

2) Find a good support group near you. Start by asking your surgeon or program coordinator.

"I am attending a support group on ______________________ (date and time) at _______________________(location)."

3) Find a few good books to read regarding the psychological and emotional issues of weight loss surgery. You can find these easily on Amazon.com.

"I have ordered and will read books titled:

____

____."

4) Consider a Lap-Band Vacation. Say the next sentences out loud.

"I am open to the idea of having my band deflated and going on healthy liquids for a few weeks. During this time, I will journal my thoughts, examine my food choices, assess why I make those food choices, and learn to meditate."

5) Research conferences for weight loss surgery patients. The support and information they provide might help you make a decision about the next step to take.

"I am going to the next ______________________________ patient conference."

Final Thoughts

"Our problems do not need to be solved. They need to be outgrown."

–Carl Jung

I feel heartbroken when a Lap-Band patient tells me that she feels like a failure because she has not been successful with her band. Usually, the patient has actually lost a fair amount of weight with the band. However, she feels unsuccessful because either she cannot lose *enough* weight or the process has been a struggle with recurrent slips, creating a cycle in which she becomes too tight, needs fluid removed and is placed on liquids for 2 weeks, is readjusted, and then reslips again. She may also feel like the weight loss has come at the cost of a normal social life. She does not know from one day to the next what she can or cannot eat or whether she will be able to go out with friends or on a date or have a lunch meeting. This creates a lot of fear and doubt and strains her relationships. Does this sound familiar?

THIS IS NOT YOUR FAULT!

It is a limitation of a tight band, and you need to know that you did nothing wrong. Please stop feeling badly about it and start taking steps to change it. First re-evaluate what you are eating to make sure you are not slipping into old bad habits; then get smarter by researching your options.

Righteous Anger: If you are not happy with your gastric band, start seeking answers, new strategies, and alternatives, like the ones found in this book. Possess a certain amount of what teenagers know inherently as righteous anger. Righteous anger is the sense that what is happening is not acceptable and that there must be something better. It can lead to a dogged determination to find a solution. Do not accept platitudes such as, "Oh, you should not be so hard on yourself...don't beat yourself up over this...we all make mistakes..." Your response needs to be, "I did not go through all of this surgery, the trouble of rearranging my life, and the process of learning new skills, just to give it all back!" Your resolution should be, "I am going to fix this!" Whether this will lead you to another surgery is uncertain, but start asking questions.

Read books, talk to your surgeon, and go back to support group. Be careful of the information you read on the Internet because weight loss revision is a personal journey, and online testimonials from well-meaning patients might not apply to your situation or suggest wrong, partial, out-of-context, or dangerous "fixes." If a physician is hesitant to give medical advice online, a total stranger is certainly not qualified to give you good advice. Medical lingo can be confusing to the untrained—it is truly a different language. I've read many online posts with poor, inflammatory, or misunderstood advice. As a bariatric surgeon, I am perplexed why my field has not become more involved in providing patient aftercare, refereeing online resources, and publishing educational materials. I hope my writings, lectures, and books help to fill this gap.

Understand that weight regain results from choices you are making, so resolve to make better choices. The choices that you make and the foods that you eat (or do NOT eat) are likely the reasons why you are regaining weight. Ask yourself, "What did diet soda ever do for me other than make me sick?" What role did chips and crackers have in your health? If it was negative, why are they back in your life? Have you not learned that dairy, cheese, chips, soda, and bread are bad for you? Perhaps the solution to your troubles could be as simple as deflating your band slightly so that you can eat fresh fruits and vegetables rather than only slider foods. If you are suffering from Mushy Food Syndrome (see Appendix D), break that cycle.

Every other "reason" is an excuse.

- Do not accept that your mother's illness is a reason to relive your childhood insecurities and start binge eating. Why not celebrate your mom's life, as opposed to lamenting her poor health?
- Do not give in to the self-loathing caused by a cheating spouse by burying your emotions in a carton of ice cream. Why not become friends with your ex-husband, as opposed to continuing to fight with him over the old furniture?
- Do not think that you are too busy with your promotion to pack a healthy lunch. Find time for the gym. Get back to the garden.
- Clear out the pantry again. What if keeping the weight off is as simple as clearing out your pantry? Instead of undergoing another surgery, why not choose to clear out the pantry once a month (or week)?
- Why not see your surgeon to make sure that everything is ok with your band instead of wondering or assuming?

Buddhist teachings tell us that:

"OBESITY IS NOTHING MORE THAN THE MANIFESTATION OF ALL OF OUR SUFFERING."

In other words, your past and present suffering shows up in your life as obesity and poor health. "Suffering" holds interesting connotations for Westerners. Often we think it implies toil, cruelty, abuse, or torture. But suffering also includes our *self-criticisms*— "I'm too fat," "I'm not good enough," or "Nobody will ever love me." Suffering can also arise from our *misperceptions*— "They are making fun of me," "He doesn't love me," or "I'm not qualified for that job." All of these thoughts can lead to obesity through self-loathing, self-dissatisfaction, or self-neglect. The older I get, the more I understand this. Stop the hurts now by letting them go. Stop the suffering by releasing the past. Forgive yourself.

Release the old labels: Think about a newborn baby. Everybody holds it and says, "She is beautiful. She is perfect." As she grows, parents (or teachers, siblings, grandparents) choose certain qualities to identify her: "This child is my athletic one...This one is my trouble-maker...My child is book-smart..."

We grow up with labels that we have allowed to define who we THINK we are. "I am shy...I am not good at math...I am a klutz...I am a carb addict...I am a chocoholic..." We often don't like them, yet we fail to realize that at ANY MOMENT we can change them. We forget that at some point in our lives,

"WE WERE ALSO THAT PERFECT BABY."

Someone held us and said, "You are perfect." At any moment, we can let the labels go and choose to be free and perfect once again.

After all, we are the highest creatures in the evolutionary chain on this planet and possibly the universe, the most divine creations of a higher power—and we cannot control ourselves around a chocolate chip cookie? Really? The psychologist Carl Jung said, "Our problems do not need to be solved. They need to be outgrown." Choose to grow up; choose to be better. The reasons that kept you obese will make you obese again, even if you do have another weight loss surgery. I see my patients outgrow their problems and change their lives everyday, so I know that you can do it too! Remember, YOU are the cannon.

Blessings to you,

Dr. V.

"Revisional surgery is a high price to pay for something that fruits and vegetables would cure." *– Dr. Vuong*

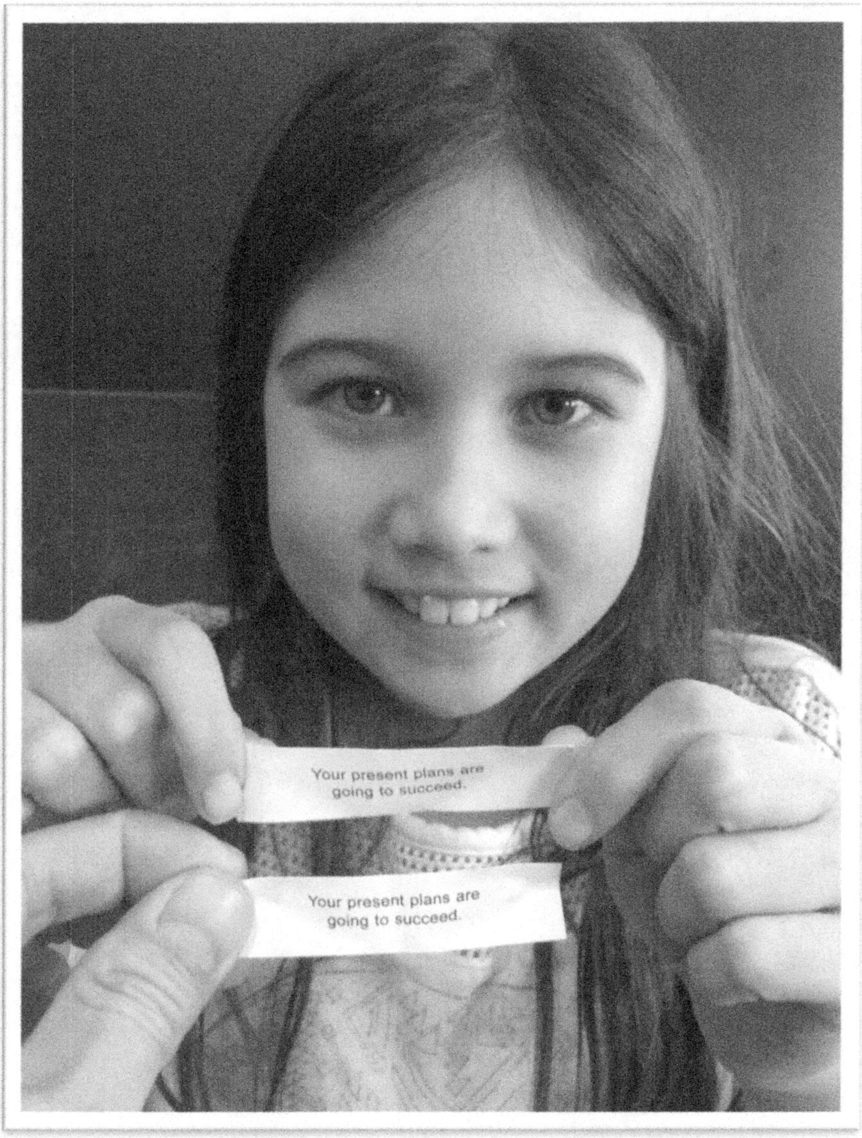

Kizzie Vuong

Notes

Appendix A: Dr. V's Formula for Success

When patients come to see me for their initial consult, I try my best to understand why and how they got to the point of needing surgery to improve their health. My background as an immigrant gives me a slightly different perspective on obesity from many healthcare professionals. In addition to my training in modern Western medicine, I bring an openness to traditional Eastern teachings. I believe that our thoughts create our reality; and it is through our thoughts that many of our illnesses manifested or worsen. Modern medicine is starting to find scientific evidence that validates many traditional Eastern teachings.

"MY BEST THINKING IS WHAT GOT ME HERE." – Alcoholics Anonymous

This teaching from Alcoholics Anonymous applies well to obesity. In fact, it applies well to all of our struggles. So where is "here?" For most of my patients, "here" is the examination table in my bariatrics clinic, talking about having 75% of their stomach removed.

If we do not want the next few years to be like the last few years, what must change? Many people will answer "my lifestyle" or "my choices." While those are true, the fundamental answer is that we must change our THINKING, because our thinking ultimately determines our lifestyle and food choices. If our best thoughts have gotten us here, all of our thoughts regarding food have basically been wrong.

If our thoughts create our reality, we should be living the life of our dreams, but instead we live in a world with a lot of suffering. If the future is to change, our thoughts must change— "I'm too fat, this cheesecake is to die for, I'm too stressed out, my husband just doesn't understand, losing weight is hard."

"You must change your mindstyle." – Dr.Vuong

Here is The Formula for Success—

Unlimited Water + Unlimited Fresh Fruits and Vegetables + Unlimited Hugs and Kisses

Unlimited Fresh Fruits and Vegetables

The key word here is *fresh.* This is the Third Rule in my clinic, or Kizzie's Rule:

YOU CAN EAT ALL OF THE FRESH FRUITS AND VEGETABLES YOU WANT, AS MUCH AS YOU WANT, ANYTIME YOU WANT.

This solves many of the common questions and struggles of weight loss surgery patients, such as,

- "What's a healthy, quick breakfast when I'm on the go?"—What could be more convenient than a banana?
- "What can I eat at my desk at work?"—How about a handful of blueberries or apple slices?
- "What can I give my kids as an afterschool snack?"— Fresh peaches or carrot sticks are great options!

The fruits and vegetables need to be fresh and mostly unadorned. For example, broccoli would be an excellent side dish, but broccoli with cheese sauce would not. Broccoli and cheese casserole transforms something healthy into something a lot less healthy. A banana is excellent, but banana bread is not. Blueberries are great, but not a blueberry muffin or blueberry Pop-Tart. And blueberries on top of your pancakes have no chance of bringing you health.

A banana is great for breakfast, and if you are still hungry after eating that banana, then have an apple, peach, or handful of blueberries. You could even have another banana if you want. And will you feel guilty if you need to have that second banana? No, of course not! Why not? Because the formula allows you to have unlimited fresh fruits and vegetables. This is key to your success—you will not feel guilty if you eat that second piece of fruit.

"THERE IS NO MORE NEED TO FEEL GUILTY WITH FOOD."

For lunch, you can have a really big salad, what my clinic calls the "Big-Ass Salad." I recommend a variety of greens—spring mixes, herb blends, kale, arugula, spinach—topped with a variety of fresh fruits and vegetables, such as tomato, bell pepper, mushrooms, beans, broccoli, and cauliflower. Add things you've never eaten before, like edamame and garbanzo beans. You can also add proteins such as couscous, tofu, fresh fish, or grilled chicken. What you top it with is not as important as the fact that the salad needs to be very large, i.e. "Big-Ass."

Hugs and Kisses

First, this means you need more literal hugs and kisses. The embarrassment about our physical size and shape that often accompanies obesity may keep us from wanting to be hugged or kissed. But we are social creatures; we are meant to touch and be touched, to love and be loved. Our souls need to be nourished by loving interactions with others. Here are some examples of how we can do more of this:

- Instead of wondering how your spouse could be with someone who has become so overweight, look at him and say, "Darling, I'm so glad you have stayed with me all of these years. We have been through so much together. You are such a blessing in my life." Don't assume he knows this just because he said, "'Til death do us part."
- Instead of complaining about why your son makes unwise choices, say to him, "Sweetie, I know you are struggling to find your way in this world, but you are my son and I will always love you and be here for you." Don't assume your child knows this because you are "Mom."
- Instead of griping about your coworker's lack of efficiency, say, "Jane, I'm here for you if you need help. Please don't hesitate to ask." Don't assume that because your cubicle is next to hers that your coworker knows you are willing to help.

In these scenarios, you may receive amazing, soul-filling hugs and kisses. And if you don't, you will probably feel better about how you are interacting with others. You will be well on your way towards reducing your anxiety and depression and increasing your health and happiness.

The "Hugs and Kisses" part of the formula also means that you must let go of the past. As much as we anguish and struggle over past events, we will never be able to change them. The past can rob you of today's happiness and hurt your chances for a bright future if you let it anger or upset you.

Patients have often told me that terrible past events caused their obesity. I'll ask, "Jane, why are you 300 pounds?" and Jane might say, "You don't know how bad I've had it...my mother was abusive; my father was an alcoholic; my son died in a car accident; my husband left me for another woman..." While those are all terrible events with undeniably lasting effects, they do not assign you to a life of continued hurt and misery. When they become excuses for becoming and staying obese, you let them continue to define who you are. Depression and anxiety are not reasons to have chips or ice cream. As difficult as it might seem, you need to let go of past hurts; otherwise, you will never be able to find peace and you will never be able to keep the weight off long term.

You might feel as though there are too many things of which you still need to let go, and you might not be sure how to do that. Let go through *forgiveness*. A powerful method for this is mirror work.

LOOK IN THE MIRROR AND SAY, "I LOVE YOU."

Notice that the formula says *nothing* about exercise or calorie counting or bad carbs or low-fat or any one of the other myriad of "tips" you have heard or tried. Nor does the formula use empty and vague phrases such as "change your lifestyle," or "make better choices." Remember, your BEST thinking is what got you here, so let go of your assumptions and acquire better information. The Formula for Success is a good place to start.

This formula is practical and easily implemented. If you start right now, it will begin working immediately. If you stop whatever you are doing right now and drink a glass of water, you will feel the results almost immediately. It does not require any new equipment or memberships. It does not require new recipes or meal plans. It does not require protein shakes or other food products that take time to ship. You can start practicing the formula right now, regardless of what you're doing, where you are in your life, or in what state your finances are.

Appendix B: The Three Rules

Rule #1: Lean protein first

- Make sure your first bite has some source of lean protein in it.
- Not "Lean protein only"
- Not "Lean protein mostly"
- Not "Lean protein always"

Rule #2: Fill your pouch with the most nutritious food you can, most of the time

- "Fill" is an imperative verb, which means it is a *command*. You must FILL your pouch with nutritious food.
- "Fill your pouch" with lean protein first, because protein keeps you full longer.
- "The most nutritious food" also means lean protein first, because if you are eating some sort of lean protein first, you are getting some sort of nutrition.
- "With nutritious foods" also means you must learn what foods are nutritious!
- The rule ends with "most of the time" because life happens. It is what you do most of the time on an everyday basis that will determine how successful you are in weight loss and in life. A meal or a day away from your plan does not mean that you have failed.

Rule #3 (Kizzie's Rule): You can eat all of the fresh fruits and vegetables you want, any time you want, as much as you want.

- Pound for pound, fresh fruits and vegetables are the most nutritious foods. Of these, leafy greens are the best.
- No one has ever said, "I'm overweight because I eat too many fruits and vegetables."
- This rule applies even if you are a diabetic.
- Canned fruits and vegetables do not count. They must be fresh!
- VARIETY provides more vitamins and minerals, so try different fruits and vegetables.

Appendix C: The Texture Scale™

Typically: Lower Nutritional Value, Lower Fat		←---IDEAL RANGE	------------→		Typically: Higher Calories, Higher Fat
1	2	3	4	5	6
Water	Mushy Foods	Fish	Shrimp/Seafood	Chicken	Steak
	Green Shakes	Fresh Fruits/Veggies		Dark White	Game Meat
	Boiled Veggies	Tofu/Egg Whites/Couscous/Quinoa		Poultry, Turkey	Pork
		Soft Salads	Tougher Salads		

- There is no limit on water.
- Bread is not on the scale because it has very little nutrition.
- Junk food, including soda, and categories labeled “carbs” or “low fat” do not appear because this is a texture scale, not a nutritional scale, though the two often overlap.
- Chips are a “liquid.” A chip will never get stuck.
- How the food item is prepared will determine where it falls on the scale.
- Reheated foods are typically thicker than when initially prepared.
- Eat between Textures 3 and 4 MOST of the time, with occasional forays into 5-6.
- Today’s mass-produced chicken is really not healthy. Neither is Turkey for that matter.
- If you lived your whole life and never ate red meat again, you’d be happier and healthier!

Appendix D: Mushy Food Syndrome

Typically:
Lower Nutritional Value
Lower Fat

Typically:
Higher Calories
Higher Fat

←---IDEAL RANGE------------→ (3 to 4)

1	2	3	4	5	6
Water	Mushy Foods	Fish	Shrimp/Seafood	Chicken	Steak
	Green Shakes	Fresh Fruits/Veggies		Dark White	Game Meat
	Boiled Veggies	Tofu/Egg Whites/Couscous/Quinoa		Poultry, Turkey	Pork
		Soft Salads	Tougher Salads		

Mushy foods—also known as slider foods—are #2 on the Texture Scale. These foods include apple sauce, mashed potatoes, refried beans, and pudding. They are typically higher in calories and lower in nutrients.

1) What will happen to your weight if you eat foods that are relatively higher in calories?

Your weight loss will plateau or you will regain weight.

2) What will your energy be like if you regularly eat foods that are typically low in nutrition?

Your energy level will be low.

3) What will your attitude be like if you have no energy?

You will have a poor attitude and probably become easily frustrated.

"Dr. Vuong, I have no energy, I am barely eating, and gosh, darn it—I'm not even losing weight!" = **Mushy Food Syndrome**

Appendix E: Protein Sources

This appendix marks a significant departure from my previous books. It is essential for our health that we start consuming more natural, non-animal-based sources of protein. (It's healthier for our planet, too.) This list is not intended to be complete, but rather to serve as an idea generator and reminder. Buy organic and locally-grown whenever possible.

BEST—EAT THESE DAILY

Vegetables—broccoli, kale, spinach

Beans—green, lima, pinto, etc. as well as lentils

Soy Products—tofu, edamame, soy milk

Whole Grains—couscous, bulgar, quinoa

Tree Nuts—almonds, cashews, walnuts; not peanut butter

Fish—fresh, preferably wild-caught, and definitely not from a can

ACCEPTABLE OCCASIONALLY

Chicken—even skinless chicken should be eaten only on occasion

Turkey—not much better than chicken

Wild poultry—quail, pheasant, duck

SAVE FOR SPECIAL OCCASIONS ONLY

Red Meat—beef is high in fat. Don't be fooled by claims that "it's a lean cut of meat." Maybe it's "leaner" than other cuts of meat, but it is still too high in fat.

Pork

Game meat—better than other meats but still high in fat

Dairy—not healthy.

> No one should drink whole milk on a daily basis, except for baby cows.
>
> Yogurt is not healthy.
>
> Choose artisanal cheeses and use them sparingly.

"Processed cheese products" have no place in anyone's diet.

Protein Supplements can be used for convenience but not regularly.

Appendix F: Super Foods

Name some Super Foods...

Apples, beans, broccoli, berries (blueberries, blackberries, strawberries, etc.), fish, lentils, kale, salad greens, seafood, spinach, tofu and other soy products, whole grains (couscous, quinoa, bulgar)

What is the difference between Super Foods and Empty Calorie Foods?

Super Foods	Empty Calorie Foods
Are ingredients	Have a list of ingredients
Come with their own packaging	Come in a package
Come from a plant	Made in a plant
Are Mother Earth-made	Are Man-made
Will spoil	Will survive a nuclear war
Will grow moldy	Mold will not eat it
Give life	Have shelf-life
Are the building blocks of our bodies	Poison us
Receive energy from the sun	Have “energy” artificially injected
Have vibrant colors that proclaim their nutritiousness	Need vibrant packaging to imitate nutritiousness
Do not have commercials	Have commercials
Make you happy	Promise happiness
Save lives	Pollute our world and our souls

Works Cited

http://www.allergan.com/Actavis/media/Allergan-PDF-Documents/Labeling/LapUS/LapBand/HM0669_L024-03_lapband_dfu.pdf

http://www.belviqhcp.com/media/1001/belviq_prescribing_information.pdf

Aarts, E.O., et al. "What happens after gastric band removal without additional bariatric surgery?" Surg Obes Relat Dis. 2014 Nov-Dec;10(6):1092-6. doi: 10.1016/j.soard.2013.10.014. Epub 2013 Oct 25.

O'Brien, PE, et al. "Long-term outcomes after bariatric surgery: fifteen-year follow-up of adjustable gastric banding and a systematic review of the bariatric surgical literature." Ann Surg. 2013 Jan;257(1):87-94

Riele, WW, et al. "Rebanding for slippage after gastric banding: should we do it?" Obes Surg. 2014 Apr;24(4):588-93. doi: 10.1007/s11695-013-1119-4.

Schauer, PR, et al. "Bariatric surgery versus intensive medical therapy for diabetes--3-year outcomes." **N Engl J Med.** 2014 May 22;370(21):2002-13. doi: 10.1056/NEJMoa1401329. Epub 2014 Mar 31.

About Dr. Duc Vuong

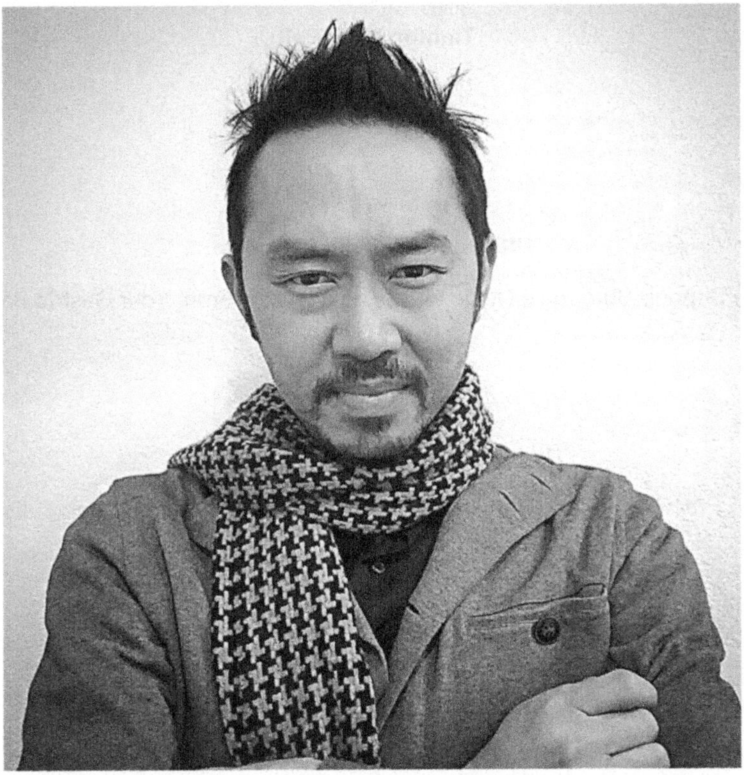

Dr. V is an internationally renowned bariatric surgeon, author, and educator. He is known as The Support Surgeon for the intensive patient educational program, which empowers his patients to change their lives. His mission is to fill the patient education gap in bariatric surgery. He does this through writing, creating videos, and utilizing social media.

Dr. V appeared in the hit TLC television show, "900 Pound Man: Race Against Time." He is currently the Director of Bariatrics at Lovelace Bariatrics in Albuquerque, New Mexico. He is a proud father, gardener, cook, and dreamer.

If you enjoyed reading this book and found it helpful, please consider leaving a review on Amazon.com. Don't forget to follow Dr. Vuong, The Support Surgeon, on Facebook for more free tips and downloads. You can also watch him on Periscope @Dr.DucVuong.

Also by Dr. Duc Vuong

Tighten Your Belt:

Overcome Obesity

Ultimate Lap-Band Success:

The Support Surgeon's Guide to Getting the Most From Your Gastric Band

Ultimate Gastric Sleeve Success:

A Practical Patient Guide to Help Maximize Your Weight Loss Results

Weight Loss Surgery Success:

Dr. V's A-Z Steps for Losing Weight and Gaining Enlightenment

Made in the USA
Monee, IL
14 September 2026

63198311R00089